TABLE OF CONTENTS

Secret Key #1 - Time is Your Greatest Enemy

Pace Yourself

Wear a watch. At the beginning of the test, check the time (or start a chronometer on your watch to count the minutes), and check the time after every few questions to make sure you are "on schedule."

If you are forced to speed up, do it efficiently. Usually one or more answer choices can be eliminated without too much difficulty. Above all, don't panic. Don't speed up and just begin guessing at random choices. By pacing yourself, and continually monitoring your progress against your watch, you will always know exactly how far ahead or behind you are with your available time. If you find that you are one minute behind on the test, don't skip one question without spending any time on it, just to catch back up. Take 15 fewer seconds on the next four questions, and after four questions you'll have caught back up. Once you catch back up, you can continue working each problem at your normal pace.

Furthermore, don't dwell on the problems that you were rushed on. If a problem was taking up too much time and you made a hurried guess, it must be difficult. The difficult questions are the ones you are most likely to miss anyway, so it isn't a big loss. It is better to end with more time than you need than to run out of time.

Lastly, sometimes it is beneficial to slow down if you are constantly getting ahead of time. You are always more likely to catch a careless mistake by working more slowly than quickly, and among very high-scoring test takers (those who are likely to have lots of time left over), careless errors affect the score more than mastery of material.

Secret Key #2 - Guessing is not Guesswork

You probably know that guessing is a good idea - unlike other standardized tests, there is no penalty for getting a wrong answer. Even if you have no idea about a question, you still have a 20-25% chance of getting it right.

Most test takers do not understand the impact that proper guessing can have on their score. Unless you score extremely high, guessing will significantly contribute to your final score.

Monkeys Take the Test

What most test takers don't realize is that to insure that 20-25% chance, you have to guess randomly. If you put 20 monkeys in a room to take this test, assuming they answered once per question and behaved themselves, on average they would get 20-25% of the questions correct. Put 20 test takers in the room, and the average will be much lower among guessed questions. Why?

1. The test writers intentionally writes deceptive answer choices that "look" right. A test taker has no idea about a question, so picks the "best looking" answer, which is often wrong. The monkey has no idea what looks good and what doesn't, so will consistently be lucky about 20-25% of the time.
2. Test takers will eliminate answer choices from the guessing pool based on a hunch or intuition. Simple but correct answers often get excluded, leaving a 0% chance of being correct. The monkey has no clue, and often gets lucky with the best choice.

This is why the process of elimination endorsed by most test courses is flawed and detrimental to your performance- test takers don't guess, they make an ignorant stab in the dark that is usually worse than random.

$5 Challenge

Let me introduce one of the most valuable ideas of this course- the $5 challenge:

You only mark your "best guess" if you are willing to bet $5 on it.
You only eliminate choices from guessing if you are willing to bet $5 on it.

Why $5? Five dollars is an amount of money that is small yet not insignificant, and can really add up fast (20 questions could cost you $100). Likewise, each answer choice on one question of the test will have a small impact on your overall score, but it can really add up to a lot of points in the end.

The process of elimination IS valuable. The following shows your chance of guessing it right:

If you eliminate wrong answer choices until only this many remain:	1	2	3
Chance of getting it correct:	100%	50%	33%

However, if you accidentally eliminate the right answer or go on a hunch for an incorrect answer, your chances drop dramatically: to 0%. By guessing among all the answer choices, you are GUARANTEED to have a shot at the right answer.

That's why the $5 test is so valuable- if you give up the advantage and safety of a pure guess, it had better be worth the risk.

What we still haven't covered is how to be sure that whatever guess you make is truly random. Here's the easiest way:

Always pick the first answer choice among those remaining.

Such a technique means that you have decided, **before you see a single test question**, exactly how you are going to guess- and since the order of choices tells you nothing about which one is correct, this guessing technique is perfectly random.

This section is not meant to scare you away from making educated guesses or eliminating choices- you just need to define when a choice is worth eliminating. The $5 test, along with a pre-defined random guessing strategy, is the best way to make sure you reap all of the benefits of guessing.

Secret Key #3 - Practice Smarter, Not Harder

Many test takers delay the test preparation process because they dread the awful amounts of practice time they think necessary to succeed on the test. We have refined an effective method that will take you only a fraction of the time.

There are a number of "obstacles" in your way to succeed. Among these are answering questions, finishing in time, and mastering test-taking strategies. All must be executed on the day of the test at peak performance, or your score will suffer. The test is a mental marathon that has a large impact on your future.

Just like a marathon runner, it is important to work your way up to the full challenge. So first you just worry about questions, and then time, and finally strategy:

Success Strategy

1. Find a good source for practice tests.
2. If you are willing to make a larger time investment, consider using more than one study guide-often the different approaches of multiple authors will help you "get" difficult concepts.
3. Take a practice test with no time constraints, with all study helps "open book." Take your time with questions and focus on applying strategies.
4. Take a practice test with time constraints, with all guides "open book."
5. Take a final practice test with no open material and time limits

If you have time to take more practice tests, just repeat step 5. By gradually exposing yourself to the full rigors of the test environment, you will condition your mind to the stress of test day and maximize your success.

Secret Key #4 - Prepare, Don't Procrastinate

Let me state an obvious fact: if you take the test three times, you will get three different scores. This is due to the way you feel on test day, the level of preparedness you have, and, despite the test writers' claims to the contrary, some tests WILL be easier for you than others.

Since your future depends so much on your score, you should maximize your chances of success. In order to maximize the likelihood of success, you've got to prepare in advance. This means taking practice tests and spending time learning the information and test taking strategies you will need to succeed.

Never take the test as a "practice" test, expecting that you can just take it again if you need to. Feel free to take sample tests on your own, but when you go to take the official test, be prepared, be focused, and do your best the first time!

Secret Key #5 - Test Yourself

Everyone knows that time is money. There is no need to spend too much of your time or too little of your time preparing for the test. You should only spend as much of your precious time preparing as is necessary for you to get the score you need.

Once you have taken a practice test under real conditions of time constraints, then you will know if you are ready for the test or not.

If you have scored extremely high the first time that you take the practice test, then there is not much point in spending countless hours studying. You are already there.

Benchmark your abilities by retaking practice tests and seeing how much you have improved. Once you score high enough to guarantee success, then you are ready.

If you have scored well below where you need, then knuckle down and begin studying in earnest. Check your improvement regularly through the use of practice tests under real conditions. Above all, don't worry, panic, or give up. The key is perseverance!

Then, when you go to take the test, remain confident and remember how well you did on the practice tests. If you can score high enough on a practice test, then you can do the same on the real thing.

General Strategies

The most important thing you can do is to ignore your fears and jump into the test immediately- do not be overwhelmed by any strange-sounding terms. You have to jump into the test like jumping into a pool- all at once is the easiest way.

Make Predictions

As you read and understand the question, try to guess what the answer will be. Remember that several of the answer choices are wrong, and once you begin reading them, your mind will immediately become cluttered with answer choices designed to throw you off. Your mind is typically the most focused immediately after you have read the question and digested its contents. If you can, try to predict what the correct answer will be. You may be surprised at what you can predict.

Quickly scan the choices and see if your prediction is in the listed answer choices. If it is, then you can be quite confident that you have the right answer. It still won't hurt to check the other answer choices, but most of the time, you've got it!

Answer the Question

It may seem obvious to only pick answer choices that answer the question, but the test writers can create some excellent answer choices that are wrong. Don't pick an answer just because it sounds right, or you believe it to be true. It MUST answer the question. Once you've made your selection, always go back and check it against the question and make sure that you didn't misread the question, and the answer choice does answer the question posed.

Benchmark

After you read the first answer choice, decide if you think it sounds correct or not. If it doesn't, move on to the next answer choice. If it does, mentally mark that answer choice. This doesn't mean that you've definitely selected it as your answer choice, it just means that it's the best you've seen thus far. Go ahead and read the next choice. If the next choice is worse than the one you've already selected, keep going to the next answer choice. If the next choice is better than the choice you've already selected, mentally mark the new answer choice as your best guess.

The first answer choice that you select becomes your standard. Every other answer choice must be benchmarked against that standard. That choice is correct until proven otherwise by another answer choice beating it out. Once you've decided that no other answer choice seems as good, do one final check to ensure that your answer choice answers the question posed.

Valid Information

Don't discount any of the information provided in the question. Every piece of information may be necessary to determine the correct answer. None of the information in the question is there to throw you off (while the answer choices will certainly have information to throw you off). If two seemingly unrelated topics are discussed, don't ignore either. You can be confident there is a relationship, or it wouldn't be included in the question, and you are probably going to have to determine what is that relationship to find the answer.

Avoid "Fact Traps"

Don't get distracted by a choice that is factually true. Your search is for the answer that answers the question. Stay focused and don't fall for an answer that is true but incorrect. Always go back to the question and make sure you're choosing an answer that actually answers the question and is not just a true statement. An answer can be factually correct, but it MUST answer the question asked. Additionally, two answers can both be seemingly correct, so be sure to read all of the answer choices, and make sure that you get the one that BEST answers the question.

Milk the Question

Some of the questions may throw you completely off. They might deal with a subject you have not been exposed to, or one that you haven't reviewed in years. While your lack of knowledge about the subject will be a hindrance, the question itself can give you many clues that will help you find the correct answer. Read the question carefully and look for clues. Watch particularly for adjectives and nouns describing difficult terms or words that you don't recognize. Regardless of if you completely understand a word or not, replacing it with a synonym either provided or one you more familiar with may help you to understand what the questions are asking. Rather than wracking your mind about specific detailed information concerning a difficult term or word, try to use mental substitutes that are easier to understand.

The Trap of Familiarity

Don't just choose a word because you recognize it. On difficult questions, you may not recognize a number of words in the answer choices. The test writers don't put "make-believe" words on the test; so don't think that just because you only recognize all the words in one answer choice means that answer choice must be correct. If you only recognize words in one answer choice, then focus on that one. Is it correct? Try your best to determine if it is correct. If it is, that is great, but if it doesn't, eliminate it. Each word and answer choice you eliminate increases your chances of getting the question correct, even if you then have to guess among the unfamiliar choices.

Eliminate Answers

Eliminate choices as soon as you realize they are wrong. But be careful! Make sure you consider all of the possible answer choices. Just because one appears right, doesn't mean that the next one won't be even better! The test writers will usually put more than one good answer choice for every question, so read all of them. Don't worry if you are stuck between two that seem right. By getting down to just two remaining possible choices, your odds are now 50/50. Rather than wasting too much time, play the odds. You are guessing, but guessing wisely, because you've been able to knock out some of the answer choices that you know are wrong. If you are eliminating choices and realize that the last answer choice you are left with is also obviously wrong, don't panic. Start over and consider each choice again. There may easily be something that you missed the first time and will realize on the second pass.

Tough Questions

If you are stumped on a problem or it appears too hard or too difficult, don't waste time. Move on! Remember though, if you can quickly check for obviously incorrect answer choices, your chances of guessing correctly are greatly improved. Before you completely give up, at least try to knock out a couple of possible answers. Eliminate what you can and then guess at the remaining answer choices before moving on.

Brainstorm

If you get stuck on a difficult question, spend a few seconds quickly brainstorming. Run through the complete list of possible answer choices. Look at each choice and ask yourself, "Could this answer the question satisfactorily?" Go through each answer choice and consider it independently of the other. By systematically going through all possibilities, you may find something that you would otherwise overlook. Remember that when you get stuck, it's important to try to keep moving.

Read Carefully

Understand the problem. Read the question and answer choices carefully. Don't miss the question because you misread the terms. You have plenty of time to read each question thoroughly and make sure you understand what is being asked. Yet a happy medium must be attained, so don't waste too much time. You must read carefully, but efficiently.

Face Value

When in doubt, use common sense. Always accept the situation in the problem at face value. Don't read too much into it. These problems will not require you to make huge leaps of logic. The test writers aren't trying to throw you off with a cheap trick. If you have to go beyond creativity and make a leap of logic in order to have an answer choice answer the question, then you should look at the other answer choices. Don't overcomplicate the problem by creating theoretical relationships or explanations that will warp time or space. These are normal problems rooted in reality. It's just that the applicable relationship or explanation may not be readily apparent and you have to figure things out. Use your common sense to interpret anything that isn't clear.

Prefixes

If you're having trouble with a word in the question or answer choices, try dissecting it. Take advantage of every clue that the word might include. Prefixes and suffixes can be a huge help. Usually they allow you to determine a basic meaning. Pre- means before, post- means after, pro - is positive, de- is negative. From these prefixes and suffixes, you can get an idea of the general meaning of the word and try to put it into context. Beware though of any traps. Just because con is the opposite of pro, doesn't necessarily mean congress is the opposite of progress!

Hedge Phrases

Watch out for critical "hedge" phrases, such as likely, may, can, will often, sometimes, often, almost, mostly, usually, generally, rarely, sometimes. Question writers insert these hedge phrases to cover every possibility. Often an answer choice will be wrong simply because it leaves no room for exception. Avoid answer choices that have definitive words like "exactly," and "always".

Switchback Words

Stay alert for "switchbacks". These are the words and phrases frequently used to alert you to shifts in thought. The most common switchback word is "but". Others include although, however, nevertheless, on the other hand, even though, while, in spite of, despite, regardless of.

New Information

Correct answer choices will rarely have completely new information included. Answer choices typically are straightforward reflections of the material asked about and will directly relate to the question. If a new piece of information is included in an answer choice that doesn't even seem to relate to the topic being asked about, then that answer choice is likely incorrect. All of the information needed to answer the question is usually provided for you, and so you should not have to make guesses that are unsupported or choose answer choices that require unknown information that cannot be reasoned on its own.

Time Management

On technical questions, don't get lost on the technical terms. Don't spend too much time on any one question. If you don't know what a term means, then since you don't have a dictionary, odds are you aren't going to get much further. You should immediately recognize terms as whether or not you know them. If you don't, work with the other clues that you have, the other answer choices and terms provided, but don't waste too much time trying to figure out a difficult term.

Contextual Clues

Look for contextual clues. An answer can be right but not correct. The contextual clues will help you find the answer that is most right and is correct. Understand the context in which a phrase or statement is made. This will help you make important distinctions.

Don't Panic

Panicking will not answer any questions for you. Therefore, it isn't helpful. When you first see the question, if your mind goes blank, take a deep breath. Force yourself to mechanically go through the steps of solving the problem and using the strategies you've learned.

Pace Yourself

Don't get clock fever. It's easy to be overwhelmed when you're looking at a page full of questions, your mind is full of random thoughts and feeling confused, and the clock is ticking down faster than you would like. Calm down and maintain the pace that you have set for yourself. As long as you are on track by monitoring your pace, you are guaranteed to have enough time for yourself. When you get to the last few minutes of the test, it may seem like you won't have enough time left, but if you only have as many questions as you should have left at that point, then you're right on track!

Answer Selection

The best way to pick an answer choice is to eliminate all of those that are wrong, until only one is left and confirm that is the correct answer. Sometimes though, an answer choice may immediately look right. Be careful! Take a second to make sure that the other choices are not equally obvious. Don't make a hasty mistake. There are only two times that you should stop before checking other answers. First is when you are positive that the answer choice you have selected is correct. Second is when time is almost out and you have to make a quick guess!

Check Your Work

Since you will probably not know every term listed and the answer to every question, it is important that you get credit for the ones that you do know. Don't miss any questions through careless mistakes. If at all possible, try to take a second to look back over your answer selection and make sure you've selected the correct answer choice and haven't made a costly careless mistake (such as marking an answer choice that you didn't mean to mark). This quick double check should more than pay for itself in caught mistakes for the time it costs.

Beware of Directly Quoted Answers

Sometimes an answer choice will repeat word for word a portion of the question or reference section. However, beware of such exact duplication – it may be a trap! More than likely, the correct choice will paraphrase or summarize a point, rather than being exactly the same wording.

Slang

Scientific sounding answers are better than slang ones. An answer choice that begins "To compare the outcomes..." is much more likely to be correct than one that begins "Because some people insisted..."

Extreme Statements

Avoid wild answers that throw out highly controversial ideas that are proclaimed as established fact. An answer choice that states the "process should used in certain situations, if..." is much more likely to be correct than one that states the "process should be discontinued completely." The first is a calm rational statement and doesn't even make a definitive, uncompromising stance, using a hedge word "if" to provide wiggle room, whereas the second choice is a radical idea and far more extreme.

Answer Choice Families

When you have two or more answer choices that are direct opposites or parallels, one of them is usually the correct answer. For instance, if one answer choice states "x increases" and another answer choice states "x decreases" or "y increases," then those two or three answer choices are very similar in construction and fall into the same family of answer choices. A family of answer choices is when two or three answer choices are very similar in construction, and yet often have a directly opposite meaning. Usually the correct answer choice will be in that family of answer choices. The "odd man out" or answer choice that doesn't seem to fit the parallel construction of the other answer choices is more likely to be incorrect.

Top 20 Test Taking Tips

1. Carefully follow all the test registration procedures
2. Know the test directions, duration, topics, question types, how many questions
3. Setup a flexible study schedule at least 3-4 weeks before test day
4. Study during the time of day you are most alert, relaxed, and stress free
5. Maximize your learning style; visual learner use visual study aids, auditory learner use auditory study aids
6. Focus on your weakest knowledge base
7. Find a study partner to review with and help clarify questions
8. Practice, practice, practice
9. Get a good night's sleep; don't try to cram the night before the test
10. Eat a well balanced meal
11. Know the exact physical location of the testing site; drive the route to the site prior to test day
12. Bring a set of ear plugs; the testing center could be noisy
13. Wear comfortable, loose fitting, layered clothing to the testing center; prepare for it to be either cold or hot during the test
14. Bring at least 2 current forms of ID to the testing center
15. Arrive to the test early; be prepared to wait and be patient
16. Eliminate the obviously wrong answer choices, then guess the first remaining choice
17. Pace yourself; don't rush, but keep working and move on if you get stuck
18. Maintain a positive attitude even if the test is going poorly
19. Keep your first answer unless you are positive it is wrong
20. Check your work, don't make a careless mistake

Identification of Infectious Disease Processes

Colonization, Infection and Contamination

Types of infection

Infection occurs when a pathogenic microorganism, such as a bacterium, invades a host of a different species and then multiplies within tissue or on the body surface, resulting in damage and/or disease.

- *Airborne infections* result from inhalation of pathogenic microorganisms (such as from dust particles) into the respiratory system.
- *Droplet/Aerosol infections* result from inhalation into the respiratory system of pathogenic microorganisms carried in droplets exhaled by others who are already infected (such as from coughing).
- *Endogenous infections* result from dormant pathogenic microorganisms reactivating within the host body (such as from tuberculosis).
- *Subcutaneous/tunnel infections* result from invasion by pathogenic microorganism of the subcutaneous tissue of an artificial opening (such as a stoma).
- *Opportunistic infections* result from pathogenic microorganisms that usually cause no infection but overgrow and invade tissue in response to suppression of the immune system from a variety of conditions, including chemotherapy, antibiotic therapy, and auto-immune disorders (such as AIDS, HIV infection).

Colonization

Colonization occurs when a pathogenic microorganism invades tissue or surface of a different species but causes either no reaction or only a slight reaction. Colonization is the first step in the infective process and usually begins with tissue in contact with the external environment and is often associated with the normal flora found on the skin. In colonization, replication does not usually occur or does not occur enough to cause infection. Colonization is present in almost all multi-cellular organisms. Colonization may be temporary or long-term and may result in the host becoming a carrier and shedding the microorganism, and thus infecting others (such as with Methicillin-resistant Staphylococcus infections—MRSA). Colonization frequently occurs in portals of entry, such as the respiratory tract, the genitourinary tract, or the gastrointestinal tract. Other common sites for colonization include the nares and axillae as well as tissues that are compromised, such as open wounds.

Contamination

Contamination is an invasion of pathogenic microorganisms into the tissue, (such as a surgical site) or onto the surface (skin) of a host or inanimate articles (such as surgical instruments or doorknobs) or substances (such as food or liquid solutions), but in fewer numbers than an infection so that there are usually insufficient numbers to cause serious compromise of tissue although contamination can result in infection. Contamination of food products with *E. coli* have caused major outbreaks of infection, so contamination can be very dangerous, and much of infection control efforts are aimed at reducing contamination of the environment in order to prevent transmission and resultant infections. A wound that is simply contaminated with a pathogenic microorganism may heal without serious problem, but if the microorganisms replicate and invade the tissue, the subsequent tissue damage may interfere with the healing process.

Occurrences, Reservoirs, and other Factors

Occurrences

Occurrences refer to the number of infectious events, both past and present, as well as the areas in which the events have occurred and the populations that have been involved.

Reservoirs are places or substances where pathogenic microorganism, such as bacteria, normally occur and multiply, depending upon this place or substance for survival. A reservoir may include an animal, a plant, a non-animate surface area, soil, or water. Usually the reservoir provides sustenance to the microorganism without compromise and allows for transmission of the microorganism to a host. Incubation periods extend from the time a pathogenic microorganism invades a host until the first signs of tissue compromise or infection occur. If the host is a vector, it is the time from invasion until first transmission to other hosts occurs. Incubation periods vary considerably, from hours to years, depending upon the type of pathogenic microorganism as well as the type of host and the environment.

Pseudo-infections and pseudo-outbreaks

Pseudo-infections should be suspected when an organism is cultured from an unusual body site or an unusual organism is cultured from any site on the body. In both cases, there is colonization of pathogens without clinical signs of infection appropriate to that organism. The colonization may be superficial, the specimen may have become contaminated, or there may have been a laboratory error. When clusters of the same type of colonization occur without infection, it is deemed a pseudo-outbreak. There are different types of pseudo-infections:
- *Pseudobacteria,* especially, *Bacillus, Pseudomonas, and Streptococcus* species, usually as the result of normal flora or contamination of the specimen.
- *Pseudomeningitis*, with bacteria or fungus in cerebrospinal fluid but without expected clinical symptoms matching the organism usually result from contamination of specimen.
- *Pseudo-pneumonias*, usually related to contaminated bronchoscopes, respiratory equipment of solutions.
- *Pseudo-bacteriuria* usually results from contamination of external urinary drainage system.

True infections must be differentiated from pseudo-infections so that patients can be properly treated.

Periods of communicability and susceptibility

Periods of communicability, also referred to as periods of infectivity, are the times after invasion of a host by a pathogenic organism during which the infectious agent can be transmitted, either directly or indirectly, to another host. Periods of communicability vary considerably, sometimes encompassing the time of incubation as well as active infection. With some types of infections, such as measles, communicability is higher during the incubation period than during the active disease. The periods of communicability may be continuous, as with HIV infection, or intermittent. Communicability/infectivity may depend upon sufficient numbers of pathogenic organisms within the blood or tissue of the host.

Susceptibility relates to a host having or lacking resistance to a particular pathogenic microorganism so that invasion results in an infectious process or disease. Susceptibility rates may vary considerably, even among the same type of hosts, depending upon such things as the time, the environment, and the state of the host's immune system.

Diagnostic findings and testing

Complete blood counts

The complete blood count with differential and platelet (thrombocyte) count provides information about the blood and other body systems and is an important part of the diagnosis of infectious processes. Red blood cell (erythrocyte) counts and concentrations may vary with anemia, hemorrhage or various disorders but are not usually an indicator of infection. Platelets may increase from a normal of 150,000-400,000 to over a million during acute infection.

White blood cell (leukocyte) count is an important indicator of bacterial and viral infection. An increase in WBCs above 10,000 mm^3 (leukocytosis) is typical of acute infections, with the amount of increase related to the severity of the infection, the age of the person, and the amount of resistance. WBC is reported as the total number of all white blood cells. Normal WBC for adults: 4,800-10,000
- o Acute infection: 10,000+; 30,000 indicates a severe infection.
- o Viral infection: 4,000 and below

Differential portion of the complete blood count
The differential provides the percentage of each different type of leukocyte. An increase in the white blood cell count is usually related to an increase in one type and often an increase in immature neutrophils, known as bands, referred to as a "shift to the left." The increase is described according to the type of cell with the primary increase, so a primary increase in lymphocytes is lymphocytosis. Before computerized reports, when laboratory slips were written by hand, the practice was to write the values for the differential from left to right in this order:
- Bands (immature neutrophils
- Segs (mature segmented neutrophils)
- Eosinophils
- Basophils
- Lymphocytes
- Monocytes

When one value increases, another decreases. With infection, the percentage of bands (the first on the left) often increases, thus resulting in the shift to the left because as the percentage of bands increases, the percentage of segmented neutrophils decreases.

The following lists the differential report for each type of white blood cell, immature neutrophils (bands), segmented neutrophils (segs), eosinophils, basophils, lymphocytes, and monocytes (expressed as a percentage of the total white blood cell (leukocyte) count):
- Normal immature neutrophils (bands): 1-3%.
  - o Increase without leukocytosis but with massive infection is a *degenerative shift.* The prognosis with this type of shift is poor because immature cells are overwhelming the blood.
  - o Increase with leukocytosis and with infection is a *regenerative shift.* The prognosis for this type of shift is good.
- Normal segmented neutrophils (segs) for adults: 50-62%.
  - o Increase with acute, localized, or systemic bacterial infection.
  - o Decrease with acute bacterial infection (poor prognosis) and viral infections.

- o Factors that affect results: stress, exercise, and obstetric labor can increase neutrophils. Steroids can affect the levels of neutrophils for up to 24 hours. Increases or decreases in eosinophils can affect percentage rate of neutrophils.
- Normal eosinophils: 0-3%.
  - o Increase than greater than 5% with allergic response and parasitic diseases.
  - o Decrease with bodily stress and acute infection.
  - o Factors that affect results: Eosinophil counts are lowest in the morning with rates rising until after midnight, so repeat tests should be done at the same time each day. Stress-inducing burns, surgery, or labor can decrease the count. Some drugs, including steroids, epinephrine, and thyroxine affect levels. Increases or decreases in basophils, monocytes, and lymphocytes affect percentage rate of eosinophils.
- Normal basophils: 0-1%.
  - o Increase with blood histamines, infection.
  - o Decrease during acute stage of infection.
- Normal lymphocytes; 25-40%.
  - o Increase in some viral and bacterial infections, such as TB.
  - o Decrease with AIDS.
- Normal monocytes: 3-7%
  - o Increase during recovery stage of acute infection.

Diagnostic equipment and procedures

X-rays are commonly used to detect infections in the lung. Chest x-rays show areas of consolidation that are often indicative of infection with purulent material present (pneumonia), especially in those with cough and fever.

Ultrasounds are especially helpful for the evaluation of cellulitis of soft tissue to determine if there is an abscess that may not be clinically evident.

Computed tomography (CT) scans may be done with fluoroscopy or contrast material, such as iodine dye, to evaluate for infections. CT scans can differentiate between cellulitis and formation of abscesses better than a routine x-ray. Chest scans can evaluate the organs and tissues of the chest for infection, abdominal scans can detect abscesses and infection, and urinary tract scans can detect infection in the kidney or bladder. A CT scan can also be used to determine the best insertion point for a needle into an abscess to effect drainage.

Magnetic resonance imaging (MRI) may be done with contrast material. It uses radio waves and magnetic fields to create images of internal structures, providing information about infections that may not be obvious with x-rays, CT scans, or ultrasounds. It is especially helpful for assessing infection of the abdominal and pelvic areas. MRIs are more expensive than x-rays, CTs, or ultrasounds so they are often done after other testing has been inconclusive.

Endoscopic procedures using a flexible endoscope inserted through the mouth (for the esophagus, stomach, and small intestine), anus (for the rectum and colon), vagina (for the vagina, cervix, and uterus), or urethra (for the urethra, bladder, and ureters), are used to visualize internal structures, such as the lining of the GI tract and the urinary tract. Endoscopes are equipped with small clippers that allow for biopsies of tissue so that it can be evaluated for infection. Endoscopes pose the risk of spreading infection.

Needle aspirations which may be completed with ultrasound or CT scan guidance, are done to aspirate serous or purulent material to relieve pressure and for culture and evaluation of infection. Needle aspirations are less invasive than biopsies and may be used with puncture wounds where there is little surface tissue loss. Multiple samples may need to be aspirated or the needle position changed, resulting in discomfort for the patient. Fine needle aspiration may be used to biopsy-infected tissue.

Biopsy of infected tissue may be done under a local anesthetic with a small amount of tissue excised to be examined microscopically, tested, and cultured. Some antiseptics like ethyl alcohol might kill the bacteria and affect resultant cultures. Biopsies may be done because visual inspection alone may not always be effective in determining if infection is present as infection may be present even without classic signs of infection, such as erythema and swelling.

Microbiology

Cultures

Cultures (in which a sample is grown on a nutrient-rich media) may be done with oxygen (aerobic) or without (anaerobic), as indicated or ordered by the physician. After the organism is cultured, sensitivity tests are usually completed to determine which anti-infective agents are most successful in treating the particular pathogenic microorganism. A Gram-stain is usually done initially, and then the culture is checked every 24 hours for colonization. Colonies are checked again with Gram-stains and also transferred to a separate media for further observation and testing. Cultures are usually negative if there is no growth in 48-72 hours unless there is a very slow-growing bacterium or fungus, which may need 4-6 weeks before final results are available. If antibiotics are begun prior to taking a sample for a culture, this can alter the results, making it very difficult to isolate the infective agent, so it's better to take a sample first and then begin antibiotics.

Types of cultures
Blood cultures, using a small sample of blood, are done to determine if an infection has invaded the bloodstream from the original site of infection, causing the infection to spread. It is also used to determine the type of bacterium or fungus and sensitivity to anti-infective agents so that proper treatment can be initiated. In many cases, if infection is present, treatment may be started before the culture results and then re-evaluated and changed as necessary when the sensitivities are complete. It is important that the skin be carefully cleansed so that the sample is not contaminated by microbes on the surface of the skin.
Wound swab cultures are done by taking swabs of wound exudate from infected tissue. The swab technique usually results in the smallest sample size so the infective agent may not grow in the culture. It is also easy to contaminate the specimen with normal bacterial skin flora.
Sputum cultures are done to determine if there is a bacterium or fungus infection of the lungs or respiratory passages. Sterile specimen containers must be used, and people must be cautioned to avoid mouthwashes that could have antiseptic properties. It's important to make sure that the specimen is coughed up and not just saliva. A sample may be obtained with a bronchoscopy as well. Viruses are frequent causes of respiratory infections, so special viral cultures, in which the sputum is mixed in a test tube with specially prepared animal cells, are often done, requiring days to weeks for final results. Various special culture procedures may be done with sputum to isolate infective agents. Cultures are not effective diagnostic tools for all types of organisms; for example, *Pneumocystis carnii*, a common cause of pneumonia in those with depressed immune system, cannot be isolated and grown in culture and must be identified by special stains.
Stool cultures are done to detect bacteria or other organisms in the stool, resulting from infection of the gastrointestinal tract. Stool samples are collected in a sterile container and must not be contaminated by toilet water or other materials, such as urine, so stools cannot be retrieved from the toilet. Stool specimens are often obtained on 3 separate days. Most intestinal infections are the result of bacteria, but fungi and viruses may also be implicated. Stool cultures are important to diagnose *Shigella Salmonella Campylobacter, Yersinia,* and *Clostridium difficile. Clostridium difficile* may result from treatment with certain antibiotics. In the case of some bacteria, such as *Clostridium difficile*, the stool culture is done to identify the particular toxin produced by a bacterium. Fungal infections, such as

Candida, may occur in those who are immune-suppressed; additionally, these same patients are also susceptible to infection with viruses, such as cytomegalovirus, so fungal and viral cultures must be done.

Antigen and antibody detection tests

Antigens are proteins of a virus or bacteria while antibodies are compounds that develop in response to antigens. Antigens are found on the surface of infective agents and antibodies in serum. A typical example of a test is the enzyme-linked immunosorbent assay (ELISA), which has an enzyme that is linked to a particular antigen or antibody so that it can detect a specific type of protein associated with the infective agent. The direct fluorescent antibodies (DFA) test uses antibodies tagged with fluorescent dye, to detect antigens. These tagged antibodies are added to a specimen and the antibodies attach to particular antigens, allowing for indirect identification when fluorescence is found upon microscopic examination. Each type of antigen has a particular shape, and only the antibodies that match that shape can attach to it, causing the fluorescent reaction and indicating that infection is present. However, some antigens have similar structure, and antibodies may attach to the wrong antigen, giving a false positive

Gram stains

Gram stain begins with mounting and fixing a specimen on a slide. The specimen is then "stained" as part of a 4-part process that uses dyes to stain Gram-positive bacteria purple and Gram-negative bacteria pink. The process must be done correctly or results can give false positives or negatives. The slide is examined microscopically for white blood cells and bacteria that indicate an infection. The size, shape, and color-stain of the bacteria help to identify it. Gram stains can be done very quickly, usually within an hour. One reason that Gram stains are done prior to cultures is to determine if the specimen is contaminated. For example, if epithelial skin cells are present in a sputum specimen, the specimen may be rejected for culture.

Gram stains during the culture procedure should use young cultures of less than 18 hours as older cultures of some Gram-positive bacteria may give the appearance of Gram-negative organisms.

Urinalysis

Urine dipstick test
The urine dipstick test for leukocyte esterase and/or nitrate is used as a quick and inexpensive test to identify purulent material or bacteria in urine. However, this test is most predictive if there are high levels of bacteria. The test for nitrate is more accurate than that for leukocyte esterase, and dipsticks that combine the two are the most accurate. While false positives are unlikely, false negatives may occur when testing for nitrates if there is diuresis that has reduced the level of nitrates in the urine, inadequate nitrates in the diet, or infections caused by *enterococci* and *acinetobacter* because these pathogens do not produce nitrates. Therefore, a high nitrate level is usually indicative of a urinary infection but the absence does not mean preclude a urinary tract infection. Because of false negatives, a negative dipstick check should be confirmed through urinalysis that includes microscopic examination in the presence of symptoms.

Diagnosis of urinary infectious processes
Urinalysis evaluates the following:
- Color is usually pale yellow/ amber and darkens when urine is concentrated, but some foods (beets) medications, stress, exercise, or excessive fluid intake may affect color. Abnormal color may be caused by blood (red), bilirubin (yellow-green), fever (dark amber/orange), or diseases (various colors).

- Appearance should be clear but may be slightly cloudy. While cloudy urine may indicate infection with pus or blood present, it can also be related to foods, vaginal contamination, and degree of hydration.
- Odor should be slight, but foods, such as asparagus and medications, such as estrogen, may affect odor. Bacteria may give urine a foul smell, depending upon the organism.
- Specific gravity is usually about 1.015 to 1.025, but may increase if protein levels increase or if there is fever, vomiting, or dehydration. Radiopaque contrast material as well as dextrose infusions may affect specific gravity.
- pH usually ranges between 4.5-8 with the average 5-6. Medications, such as Mandelamine, some foods, such as cranberries, and Vitamin C may make urine acid (less than 7 pH). An alkaline urine (above 7) occurs with bacteriuria, urinary tract infections, as well as kidney and respiratory diseases.
- Sediment is examined microscopically: *Red cell casts* from acute infections, *broad casts* from kidney disorders, and *white cell casts* from pyelonephritis. *Leukocytes* > 10 per ml^3 are present with urinary tract infections. Crystals should be absent.
- Glucose, ketones, protein, blood, bilirubin, and nitrate should be negative. Urobilinogen should be 0.1-1.0 units. Urine glucose may increase with infection (with normal blood glucose). Frank blood may be caused by some parasites and diseases but also by drugs, smoking, excessive exercise, and menstrual fluids. Increased red blood cells in the urine may result from infections of the lower urinary tract.

Urine culture and sensitivities

Urine culture and sensitivities are done to identify infective agents. Results should show fewer than 10,000 organisms/ ml of urine. Bacteria found are the result of pathogenic microorganisms or contamination from skin. Counts higher than 10,000 are considered diagnostic for infection. Urine is easily contaminated if clean catch procedures are not followed carefully and if people have poor hygiene. Urine may be too dilute for accurate culture if patients have a large fluid intake. Urine left at room temperature may begin to grow organisms so the results are not accurate. Urine should not be refrigerated more than 2 hours before testing. Urine intended for testing for cytomegalovirus must not be refrigerated. Urinary cultures are positive for urine infection if the organism is found on Gram stain and if two urine cultures isolate the same organism with >102 colonies/ml of urine in catheterized specimens or <105 colonies/ml of urine with patients receiving appropriate antibiotics.

Immunity and Immunizations

Immunity to infectious diseases is acquired through vaccinations or antibodies in response to a natural infection. Immunity with vaccinations usually takes 10-14 days, but the length of time varies according to the type of vaccination. Immunity may be almost 100% or much lower, again depending upon the type of vaccination and the disease. Natural infections do not always confer immunity, and there is no immunity for some infections, such as HIV. Most people who went to school in the United States received vaccinations as children in order to attend school.

Hepatitis B

Health care providers who contact blood or body fluids should be immunized for hepatitis B. The anti-Hbc test can identify people who were previously vaccinated or infected with hepatitis B and may have acquired immunity or the chronic form of the disease. Those who test positive for anti-HBc, must also be tested with HBsAg to determine if they have chronic infection rather than immunity.

Tuberculosis

Immunity to tuberculosis (TB) is established by regular 1-2 times yearly TB testing, most often with a tuberculosis skin test (TST), or with the QuantiFERON®-TB Gold test, which uses whole blood to test for *Mycobacterium tuberculosis,* including both latent and active infection although it cannot differentiate the two. Positive tests are followed by chest x-rays, sputum cultures, and clinical evaluation. BCG (bacille Calmette-Guérin) is a tuberculosis vaccine routinely administered to children in countries with high incidences of childhood tuberculous meningitis. It is not recommended in the United States because infection with *Mycobacterium tuberculosis* has a low incidence and adult immunization is variable. QuantiFERON®-TB Gold test is not affected by prior BCG vaccination but TST can show false positives. Health care workers may receive BCG vaccinations if they work with a large number of TB patients with resistant strains of TB, there is ongoing transmission of this disease to healthcare workers, and TB control precautions are unsuccessful.

Measles, mumps, and rubella (MMR) and influenza

Most children are now immunized against measles, mumps, and rubella through the MMR vaccination at about 12-15 months, and many adults have developed immunity through naturally acquired infections. Serological testing for rubella should be done for women of childbearing age so they can be offered vaccinations before becoming pregnant. Women should avoid pregnancy for at least 8 weeks after a vaccination. Healthcare workers who do not have immunity and are pregnant should not be assigned to work with patients who may have rubella. Non-immune adults may receive MMR.

Influenza strains vary from year to year and the only way to insure that immunity is current is for people to receive yearly influenza vaccinations that provide protection against the influenza virus. Vaccines are composed about 6 months before flu season each year, so some viruses that arise after that time may not be included in the vaccine.

Active and passive immunization

Active immunization utilizes antigens from parts of the infectious pathogen (acellular vaccines), attenuated (weakened) live organisms from disease-causing pathogens, or bacterial toxins treated with chemicals to cause the body to develop antibodies or T lymphocytes against the disease. Some vaccinations provide lifetime immunity but others lesson the severity of disease. Other vaccinations, such as tetanus, require boosters at particular intervals. Because active immunization contains antigens, they may put people who are immunosuppressed, such as those with AIDS or who are on immunosuppressive drugs or chemotherapy, at risk for contracting the disease.

Passive immunization utilizes antibodies, immune globulin, from another person or animal that was actively immunized against a disease. These antibodies survive for about 14-21 days, conferring temporary resistance to a disease. One advantage to passive immunization is that it provides protection right away. Immune globulin derived from animals, such as horses, poses more of a potential for adverse allergic reactions than human-derived immune globulin.

Epidemiologic markers for bacteria

Outbreak investigations occur when a pattern of infection occurs, suggesting a single causative agent. It is necessary to isolate the microorganism and to differentiate it from other strains in order to determine if there is an actual outbreak. In some cases, an outbreak may be related to an increase in resistance rather than an increase in infection rates, and this needs to be determined as well.

Traditionally, *phenotyping,* which studies the appearance of the microorganism or the reactions, was done to identify epidemic strains. Phenotyping includes identification of the genus, species, biotype, serotype, and phage type. Phenotyping determines the genetic traits of the microorganism, but some microorganisms share the same or similar phenotypic markers, making it difficult to distinguish each strain of a particular species. Additionally, random mutations may occur. Newer techniques of molecular strain identification involve *genotyping,* which studies the composition of the DNA/RNA of microorganisms. Typing can differentiate strains and determine if they are indistinguishable.

Biotyping

Biotyping involves identifying different biochemical reactions. There are multiple methods, such as identifying the ability of a microorganism to ferment sugars. There are kits available for typing of different microbes; however, biotyping does a poor job of distinguishing among strains.

Bacteriophage typing

Bacteriophage typing uses bacteriophages, which are viral intracellular parasites with the ability to infect bacteria by entering, multiplying, and destroying (lysing) the cell. A series of bacteriophages with different ability to lyse a cell is used to differentiate strains of bacteria, depending upon the microorganism's susceptibility to lysis. This technique is time-consuming and not widely available because stocks of phages must be maintained. This test is most useful for identify *staphylococcus* strains. It has been replaced by DNA based genotyping methods.

Bacteriocin typing

Bacteriocin typing involves the identifying different antibacterial toxins that are produced by an individual strain of bacteria. This method is rarely used nowadays.

Protein typing

Protein typing determines differences in proteins made by strains of bacteria.

Antimicrobial susceptibility testing

Antimicrobial susceptibility testing uses *in vitro* (test tube or agar) testing of microorganism's susceptibility to antibiotics to predict how successful antimicrobials will be in the body. The test measures how much an organism grows or multiplies when subjected to various antimicrobials in order to provide information to guide in the selection of appropriate treatment.

In a typical test, bacteria are swabbed on an agar plate and then small antibiotic-impregnated paper disks with different antibiotics are placed in a circle around the disk over the bacteria. The plate is incubated and then the area where growth of bacteria has been inhibited is measured to determine the "zone of susceptibility." That is if there is a large area with inhibited growth, the microorganism is considered *susceptible.* If there is no zone of inhibition or very little, the microorganism is considered *resistant.* Some microorganisms show incomplete susceptibility and are considered *intermediate.*

Restriction endonuclease analysis

Restriction endonuclease analysis uses restriction enzymes to identify bacterial strains. Restriction enzymes are particular bacterial proteins that recognize unique chromosomal DNA and plasmids, which are circular, double strands of DNA that can replicate in a cell but are separate from chromosomal DNA. Restriction enzymes cleave (split) the DNA at specific sequences. The fragments that are cleaved can be separated by size to produce a *restriction endonuclease profile.* This method can detect small differences in bacterial strains. There are 3 different types of restriction enzymes that can be used:

- Type 1 can recognize unique chromosomal DNA but cleaves the strand at random at least 1000 base pairs (bp) from the site that they recognize.
- Type II, the most commonly used restriction enzyme in recombinant DNA methods, recognizes the unique site and cleaves at that point, producing predictable strands.
- Type III also recognize the unique chromosomal DNA but cleave at least 25 bps away. This method is useful for bacteria, viruses, and parasites that don't have plasmids

Pulsed-field gel electrophoresis (PFGE)

Pulsed-field gel electrophoresis (PFGE) is a method of typing that separates large DNA strands. A typical technique is to apply 3 pairs of electrodes to a gel plate to which large DNA, produced by restriction enzymes that break the DNA into small numbers of large DNA fragments. The plate is covered with dye. A current that changes directions in a regular pattern is applied to the gel until the dye has spread across the gel. Then a solution is added that binds to DNA and causes it to fluoresce. Changing the direction of the current allows smaller DNA fragments to move more quickly than larger fragments so there is separation of long and short strands, providing the typical DNA band profile. Different organisms have different band patterns. Organisms are considered distinguishable if there have more than three bands in different positions. This typing method is very accurate, especially for *staphylococci, enterococci,* and *P. aeruginosa.*

Plasmid profile analysis

Plasmid profile analysis involves the development of a plasmid profile. Plasmid DNA is isolated from a microorganism, and then the plasmid DNA is separated by agarose gel electrophoresis. Plasmids can spread from one species or strain to another through process called conjugation, so in some instances, an outbreak can be traced to plasmids rather than to a bacterial strain. However, this mobility of plasmids interferes with analysis. Analysis is improved by using restriction endonuclease enzymes to digest the plasmids and create fragments that are then analyzed by electrophoresis. Plasmid profile analysis can be applied to many different bacterial strains and can be completed within one day, but epidemic strains may not contain plasmid or strains that aren't part of the epidemic may contain the same plasmid profile as the epidemic strains. So, while plasmid profile analysis is a rapid and inexpensive technique for typing, it is not always accurate or sufficient.

DNA hybridization

DNA hybridization, or genetic probing, involves a process in which DNA is denatured, heated to a temperature that allows the DNA to form into single strands. As the DNA is cooled, it recoils and can be joined to a complementary probe of labeled DNA (usually with radioactive phosphorous), forming a hybrid, which is measured. Essentially a DNA, or sometimes RNA, strand is marked chemically or radioactively with a substance that will bind to a particular gene, allowing this gene to be identified and isolated. This typing technique can profile similarities in sequence among various DNAs as well as the repetition of sequence in one DNA. Genetic probing is used to find specific fragments of DNA, referred to as target DNA. This form of typing does not require a viable pathogen and can identify individual strains of bacteria. It can also identify pathogens, such as rotavirus, and chlamydia, which are difficult to cultivate; however, it is a slow process and often not as sensitive as cultures.

Ribotyping

Ribotyping is a type of DNA fingerprinting analysis that utilizes genes that provide code for ribosomal ribonucleic acids (rRNA). Various proteins along with ribosomal RNA comprise the ribosome, which is a structure within the cell in which proteins are manufactured. The ribosome uses coding from the rRNA to place the correct amino acids in proteins. The genetic coding for rRNA varies more between bacterial strains than within them, so ribotyping distinguishes between bacterial strains. Restriction enzymes are used to cleave the genes that code for the rRNA into fragments, and then electrophoresis is used to separate the fragments. Genetic probes are used to highlight fragments of different sizes so that they appear as bands in the profile. Different ribotypes have banding patterns that correspond to each type. Ribotyping has been successful in typing a variety of microorganisms, including strains of *Salmonella typhi, E. coli, Campylobacter, Pasteurella multocida,* and various forms of *staphylococcus.*

Polymerase chain reaction (PCR)

Polymerase chain reaction makes millions of replications of specific DNA sequences without a living microorganism. When cells divide naturally, polymerase enzymes copy the DNA found in each chromosome by separating the two strands of the DNA helix, so each strand can be copied and then replicated. This process also requires the 4 nucleotide bases. Additionally a short sequence of nucleotide, primase, called a "primer" is needed to begin the replication process. This can be done within a test tube, which is heated to separate the DNA strands, then cooled so the primer can begin the process, and heated again so that the polymerase can begin to make copies using the nucleotides. This 2-hour method can be used to replicate and detect more than 22 different microorganisms that fail to grow well or at all in cultures. It can detect coding genes for toxins, virulence and antimicrobial resistance, making this an effective tool for infection control.

Sentinel events

Sentinel events are defined by the Joint Commission as a death or serious physical injury that is unexpected. This death or injury could be related to many things, including surgery on the wrong body part, suicide, or infection. With infections, it is considered a sentinel event if it is determined that the death or injury would not have occurred without the infection. Each case must be dealt with individually, and, if defined as sentinel, a *root cause analysis* that defines the problem through gathering evidence to identify what contributed to the problem must be done. Once a root cause has been determined, an *action plan* that identifies all the different elements that contributed to the problem is recommended and instituted. The theory is that finding the root cause can eliminate the problem rather than just treating it. Thus, finding the source of an infection would be more important than just treating the infection.

Epidemiologically significant organisms

Epidemiologically significant organisms are those with potential to cause death or serious injury or disease. Some organisms are considered significant because they are invasive and cause outbreaks but also are often resistant to antimicrobials, making control difficult. When epidemiologically significant organisms are identified, usually through active surveillance or cultures, enhanced infection control methods may be needed to control spread of the infection. Microorganisms that are significant include vancomycin-resistant *enterococci* (VRE), *Clostridium difficile* that has caused infection, methicillin-resistant *Staphylococcus aureus (MRSA)* as well as others that can be transmitted directly or indirectly. Antibiotic resistance is increasing among gram-negative bacilli such as *Klebsiella pneumoniae, P. aeruginosa,* and *Enterobacter* spp. Organisms that are deemed significant may vary from one department to another, so that organisms that might prove fatal in the neo-natal unit may pose less of a threat to adults, but a facility must be viewed as one unit because of the potential for spread of infection.

Collection, handling, transport, and storage techniques

Urine specimens

Urine specimens should be collected following standard procedures.
- *Specimen containers* should hold at least 50 ml and have a wide base. They should be sterile, leak resistant, break proof, and have a secure lid. Containers are used only one time and then discarded with other biohazard material.
- *Collection* may be from straight catheterization, drainage from a Foley catheter, or obtained for urination. The staff handling the container and the patient instructed in proper method for obtaining the specimen should wear gloves. The containers should be labeled properly, not on the lid, which might become separated from the container.
- *Transport* should be with the specimen container inside of a second container, such as a Ziploc bag so that urine that might be on the outside of the container doesn't spread contamination.
- *Storage* should be in a designated area and inside the transport container.

Swabs

Swabs may be used to collect specimens from the nares, the throat, or wounds. If purulent material is being collected from a wound, it is better to send a sample of the pus in a sterile container rather than collecting a specimen with a swab if the drainage is sufficient.
- *Collection* should be done wearing gloves and holding the container that receives the swab as close as possible to the swabbed area to avoid contaminating the environment with droplets. The container should be labeled before collection. The swab is inserted into the container, usually a tube, slowly to avoid contaminating the mouth. Some types require that the end of the swab be broken or cut, which has the potential for spreading infection, so this should be done gently,
- *Handling* the specimen container should be after the container is bagged.
- *Transport* should be done immediately.
- *Storage* should be in designated areas following guidelines.

Sputum

Sputum specimens can easily contaminate the outside rim of the container as people often cough directly over the container or place their mouths on it, so containers should always be considered contaminated.
- *Collection* should be done wearing gloves if obtaining the specimen directly from the patient and when handling the container. If the patient collects the specimen, the patient should be instructed how to do so. The container should be wide-mouthed and hold at least 50 ml. If possible, the rim should be wiped before the lid is applied and the tissue placed in the biohazard

waste receptacle. Collection should be done outside, at a distance from other people, and not in the laboratory.

- *Handling* should be minimal. The specimen container should be placed inside a Ziploc bag that is labeled with name, date, and time of collection.
- *Transport to* the lab should be done immediately.
- *Storage* should be in designated areas following guidelines.

Aspirants

Aspirants include any fluids aspirated from the chest, joints, cerebrospinal area, sinuses, abscesses, cysts, or other.

- *Collection* requires aseptic techniques, including gloves, with needle puncture and then aspiration of fluid. Skin antiseptics are used, but those with a strong residual effect, such as chlorhexidine, should be avoided. The container should be dry, break-proof, and sterile. A protective mask is usually not needed although it may be used when obtaining cerebrospinal fluid with some infectious diseases, such as meningococcal meningitis. The needle should be removed if there is a safety method to prevent needle stick in order to reduce spraying and the fluid gently expelled into the specimen container, which is then bagged.
- *Handling* should be with gloves until the container is bagged.
- *Transport* to the lab should be done immediately.
- *Storage* should be in designated areas following guidelines specific for the type of aspirant. Cerebrospinal fluid degrades quickly and should be tested immediately.

Fecal specimens

Fecal specimens should not be contaminated with urine, paper, or toilet water, especially if they are to be examined for microorganisms.

- *Collection* should be done after the patient has urinated, if possible the specimen can be collected in a clean bedpan. Plastic wrap is sometimes placed over the back part of the toilet to catch the feces, but the plastic can become easily contaminated. The fecal specimen is placed in a sterile container, preferably one with a scoop in the lid to facilitate transfer. About 10 mls should be collected for viral or bacterial testing. Testing for parasites requires a larger specimen. The person handling the container and specimen should wear gloves. Swabs of fecal material are almost never sufficient for adequate testing.
- *Handling* should be done after specimen container is bagged with label indicating, name, date, and time of collection.
- *Transport* should be done as quickly as possible.
- *Storage* should be in designated areas following guidelines.

Blood

Blood should always be considered hazardous and potentially infectious.

- *Collection* should be done using antiseptic techniques and sterile equipment with the person collecting wearing gloves. Collection should be done using vacuum tube blood collection devices. Avoid the use of needle syringes if possible, or if blood must be transferred from the syringe care should be used to avoid spraying blood or leaking droplets. In some cases, protective eyewear may be used. Blood should not be collected from an arm into which IV fluids are being administered as this can dilute the sample. Blood is drawn in a particular order if multiple tubes are used so that there is no cross-contamination with additives.

- *Handling* should include mixing the additive with the blood by rotating the tubes.
- *Transport* to the laboratory should be done immediately.
- *Storage* should be in designated areas following guidelines for the type of testing that is to be done.

Antimicrobials and Microbiologic Monitoring

Prophylactic antimicrobial therapy refers to treatment prior to infection in order to prevent an infection from occurring. Prophylaxis has been over-used and inconsistent and has contributed to antibiotic resistance, so duration should be short and the need should be evaluated individually, following guidelines that have been established to provide optimal benefit.

Empiric antimicrobial therapy refers to beginning treatment when an infection appears clinically obvious but the specific causative agent has not yet been identified, such as when a person has pneumonia. Empiric therapy should be given following guidelines and recommendations that consider the site of infection, the most like causative agents, hospital epidemiology, cost, and susceptibilities.

Therapeutic antimicrobial therapy refers to using treatment that is appropriate for particular microorganisms, following guidelines that have been established in relation to diagnosis, causative agent, cost, and susceptibilities. Treatment should be neither too broad nor narrow and of sufficient duration.

Recommendations

The National Surgical Infection Prevention Project has issued recommendations for the use of preoperative antimicrobial prophylaxis. General recommendations include:
- *Timing:* The first dose should be administered within 1 hour of incision. If a fluoroquinolone or vancomycin is indicated, then it should be administered within 2 hours of incision.
- *Duration:* Antimicrobials for most procedures should end within 24 hours of surgery.
- *Limiting additional antimicrobials:* Pre-existing infections should be treated prior to surgery whenever possible. If not, then additional antimicrobial, specific to existing infection, may be necessary.
- *Dosing:* Dosage should be based on age and weight, according to recommendations. Lengthy surgeries may require additional intraoperative dosing.
- *Providing alternatives for those with allergies:* Patients with confirmed allergies to commonly used prophylactic agents would need an alternative antimicrobial. Clindamycin and vancomycin can be considered if data shows the facility does not have a problem with resistance or incidences of infection with *Clostridium difficile* or *Staphylococcus epidermis.*

Microbiologic Monitoring

Environmental microbiologic monitoring involves ensuring that housekeeping staff maintains a clean environment, but routine sampling of walls, floors, other surfaces, and air in a medical institution is usually not indicated unless an outbreak presents, as the environment is rarely the cause of infection except in those who are immunocompromised. Studies have shown that visual assessment of cleanliness is not always supported by testing. A quick test for contamination is the *adenosine triphosphate bioluminescence test*; however, finding large numbers of organisms is common, depending upon the number of people in a room, activity, airflow, and other factors. Total bacterial counts generally do not correlate with infection risk. Valid testing requires cultures and quantitative results, with results reported as the number of organisms per area or volume so that swabbing a large area is not compared to swabbing a small area. Sampling methods may include swabbing with a moist sterile swab, a moist gauze, or HEPA vacuum sock. Dry swabs are less efficient at identifying spores.

Assessment of Patient and Employee Status

Signs and symptoms of infections

Patients
Signs and symptoms of infection in patients should be assessed continually. Common infections involve the wound or surgical site, the lungs, and the urinary system, so particular attention should be paid to these areas. Assessment will vary according to diagnosis:
- Wound or surgical site should be checked and evaluated for erythema, edema, and discharge.
- Systemic indications of infection, such as an increase in temperature or changes in vitals signs should be monitored regularly.
- Lungs should be evaluated by spirometer and auscultation. Cough, shortness of breath, or sputum production should be noted. Patient should receive instruction in deep breathing and coughing exercises to prevent atelectasis.
- Urine should be monitored for amount, color, and consistency and any burning or other dysuria should be evaluated. Discomfort in the bladder area, flanks, or lower back could indicate infection. Ensuring adequate fluid intake and monitoring intake and output can help to prevent urinary infections.

Employees
Signs and symptoms of infection in employees should be discussed as part of inservice so that employees know the type of symptoms that they should report for potential laboratory confirmation and those for which they should not report to work because of the danger they pose to others. For example, a person with a cough, an active infection, or diarrhea should not work with patients. Additionally, those with open cuts or rashes, such as from eczema, that compromise the integrity of the skin or at higher risk for developing skin infections, such as *staphylococcus aureus,* which may not be obvious at first. Employees should be tested for immunity to infectious diseases and immunized before coming in contact with patients as this will reduce the incidence of infection, but immunity is not possible for all conditions, so infection control policies that are clear and effective are critical.

Exposure to communicable disease

Patients
Patient exposure to communicable disease can be difficult to assess as the person may not be aware of exposure or may be reluctant to discuss it because of privacy issues. Doing a careful and thorough history and physical assessment can provide information that suggests exposure. Questioning people about symptoms rather than diseases may elicit more information: "Have you had contact with anyone with a rash?" or "Have you experienced night sweats?" Exposure to a communicable disease can occur outside of the hospital as well as inside. Exposure to communicable disease can be endogenous (self-infection) or exogenous (cross-infection). Endogenous infections, for example, can result from the normal body flora or an area of infection (such as a boil) contaminating a surgical wound. Exogenous infections can occur by contact with someone who is infected, such as another patient or staff member, or by airborne particles. Both types of infection can occur in the hospital.

<u>Employees</u>

Employees in a medical facility are exposed to communicable diseases on a regular basis. Any droplets from cough or contact with bodily fluids has the potential for exposing an employee to infection, so employees must always be alert to possible exposure. Employees should wear gloves when handling any types of bodily fluids, including urine and feces. Universal precautions should be used by all staff with patient contact. Any contact with blood should be considered as potentially infective and should be reported. Needlestick policies should be in place to determine what type of laboratory tests or prophylaxis will be administered. Control of exposure is best done through immunity, so all employees should fill out comprehensive histories and be required to have routine immunizations so that exposure does not result in transmission of infection. Handwashing procedures should be reviewed regularly and hand sanitizers should be available in all patient's rooms as this is an effective method of reducing exposure and transmission.

Bloodstream infections

Bloodstream infections (BSI) have increased markedly over the last few decades with approximately 350,000 patients infected each year. BSI are defined as pathogens isolated in the blood of someone hospitalized for >48 hours. There are 2 basic types:
- *Primary* infections arise in the bloodstream and may be related to intravascular devices.
- *Secondary* infections spread systemically from an infection elsewhere in the body, such as from a urinary or wound infection.

There are a number of issues related to diagnosing a BSI from blood cultures:
- *Skin preparation* must be adequate to prevent contamination of sample.
- *lood volume* must be 10-20 ml in order to detect low concentrations of organisms.
- *Timing* should be as soon as possible after symptoms appear.
- *Venipuncture* should be done peripherally rather than obtaining blood from intravascular catheter, which may be contaminated.

Risk factors

Surgical site infections: There are a number of risk factors that are associated with increased rates of hospital-acquired surgical site infections:
- *Length of hospitalization* prior to surgery beyond 1 day increases risk. Studies have shown that infection rates more than double by 1 week preoperative stay.
- *Razor shaves* cause small cuts that can markedly increase the danger of infection to 20% if done 24 hours before surgery. Shaving with an electric shaver or using a depilatory have lower rates of infection, and no hair removal at all has the lowest rate.
- *Operative time*, especially beyond 2 hours, increases infection rates.
- *Remote infections* increase risk by over 2.5 times.
- *Surgeon skill* can affect risk; more experienced surgeons tend to have lower infection rates.
- *Surgical drains* have been implicated in some studies but not others.
- *Host factors* such as age, diabetes, and immunosuppression can increase risk. Obesity is also associated with increased risk.

Transmission

Patients or staff with suspicious symptoms, such as an unexplained or chronic cough or foul discharge, should be monitored carefully and appropriate lab testing and precautions taken to reduce the risk of transmission. Most infections are not easily transmissible, but those in close contact with an infected person have some risk. Prophylaxis may be needed to protect staff and other patients if there is substantial risk of transmission. There are a number of factors that increase risk of transmission to both staff and employees:

- Patient beds in very close proximity, less than 1 meter, increase the chance of cross infection.
- Sharing of equipment among different patients can spread microorganisms.
- One employee making contact with multiple patients increases the chance of cross infection.
- Failure to use adequate handwashing procedures and universal precautions increases the chance of transmitting infection.
- Inadequate monitoring of infections and lab reports can lead to outbreaks.

Laboratory results

Laboratory results for patients should be evaluated on a daily basis, at least, to check for any organisms that might spread or cause an outbreak"

- *Streptococcus pyogenes*
- *Staphylococcus aureus*
- Vancomycin-resistant enterococci
- *Shigella spp.*
- *Salmonella* spp.
- *Mycobacterium tuberculosis*
  Pseudomonas aeruginosa
- *Neisseria meningitidis*
- *Legionella* spp.

Additionally, organisms that might pose particular problems to certain patient populations, such as in the neo-natal unit, should be flagged for evaluation. Staff must be alert to the possibility of infection so that cultures or other laboratory tests can be done if there is a suspicion of an infection because lab reports alone are insufficient as some infections may be present without lab tests. Staff with signs of infection or possible exposure should be sent for appropriate lab testing and relieved of work duties if there is likelihood that they pose a risk to patients or other staff.

Host risk factors

Host risk factors are those conditions or circumstances that put the host at increased risk of developing an infection. Host risk factors include the following:

- *Age:* Those who are very young or very old are often at increased risk. Infants may not have developed antibodies, and the elderly may have decreased immunity.
- *Disease:* Many diseases, such as diabetes and leukemia, increase the risk of infection.
- *Circulatory impairment:* Any decrease in perfusion to an area from disease or injury increases the chance of infection.
- *Medications:* Immunosuppressants and chemotherapy can reduce immunity. Improper use of antibiotics builds resistance.
- *Contact:* Close contact with the source of microorganisms increases the host risk factor.
- *Wounds and instrumentation:* Surgical wounds, ulcers, catheters, or any other thing that allows microorganisms easy access increases risk.
- *sence of prophylactic antibiotics:* Antibiotics have proven to reduce risk of post-operative infections for some procedures, but guidelines for use are not always followed.

Pathogenesis and Classification

Stages

Pathogenesis is the cellular responses and other pathological events involved in the infectious process. A pathogenic organism must find a means of *transmission* from a reservoir to gain access to the host. Once entry is achieved, in order to grow and replicate, the microorganism must attach, through a mechanism called *adherence*, so that it can become established within the host. Some will then use adhesins to attach to a cell for the purpose of entering inside of the cell. This can cause infection of just one type of cell or, in some cases, generalized infection. Microorganisms can cause localized infection, but some emit toxins that can cause disseminated or distant infection or cell damage. Microorganisms *produce* a variety of chemicals, including toxins, to help them gain control. The invading microorganism must *evade* the immune system, which mounts a defence to protect the body. Once entrenched, the microorganism then *transmits* to a new host.

Transmission and virulence

Transmission can often be evaded by the host if the skin is intact and the mucosa is healthy. Normal flora usually remains in balance unless disease or medications affect the immune system. Pathogenic microorganisms, however, have developed numerous strategies to invade a host. Some spores can withstand long periods in the environment and are resistant to heat and drying, some organisms thrive on the skin and can easily spread to wounds, some can survive well in contaminated fluids, others thrive in conditions of poor hygiene. Incision, rashes, tubes, or trauma that compromises the integrity of the skin or mucous membranes facilitates transmission.

Virulence is the degree of pathogenicity, the ability to cause infection in the host. When comparing organisms, virulence is often evaluated in terms of the infectious/effective dose (ID50/ED50) that will likely cause infection in 50% of those exposed or the lethal dose (LD50) that will cause death in 50% of those exposed.

Virulence factors, which allow the microorganism to invade a host and multiply, vary from one microorganism to another, with some much more virulent than others because of inherent characteristics:
- Adherence: Some bacteria are more readily able to adhere to mucosal surfaces, such as those that develop fimbriae that facilitate adherence, making them more able to colonize and multiply.
- Invasiveness: Some bacteria have chemical components on their surfaces, either on the plasmids or chromosome, which facilitate invasion of host cells.
- Structure: Some bacteria are encapsulated, effectively protecting them from phagocytosis or destruction.
- Toxins: Many bacteria produce lipopolysaccharide, protein, or enzyme toxins (endotoxins and exotoxins) that are extremely poisonous to the host and can cause severe systemic reactions, acute infection, sepsis, shock, and death.
- Iron-biding factors (siderophores): Some bacteria are able to use the host's supply of iron to multiply and grow, competing with the host and facilitating infection.

Types of infections

Bacterial infections include:
- *Subclinical* causes no obvious symptoms

- *Latent* occurs when people have no symptoms of infection but can be carriers.
- *Accidental* occurs outside of the normal transmission mode, such as from needle sticks or acts of bioterrorism.
- *Opportunistic* occurs when normal flora overgrows, usually in the presence of immunosuppression.
- *Primary* includes clinical symptoms.
- *Secondary* follows a primary infection because of host compromise.
- *Mixed* occurs when more than one pathogen is the causative agent.
- *Acute presents* rapidly with obvious symptoms that may persist for days or weeks.
- *Chronic* persists for long periods of time, months or years.
- *Localized* remains in a circumscribed area.
- *Systemic* is generalized and may involve many different areas of the body, often spread through the blood stream.
- *Retrograde* is that in which the bacteria are able to ascend a structure, such as a duct.
- *Fulminant* is severe, rapid, acute infections.

Symbiotic relationships

Microorganisms have three types of relationships with humans: *mutualism*, *commensalism*, and *parasitism*. Symbiotic relationships involve two organisms living together. Symbionts spend all or part of their lives living in association with an organism of a different species.

Mutualism includes a mutualist and a host. Both benefit because they have a metabolic dependence upon each other, in some cases with the host providing necessary nutrients for the mutualist. The E. coli in the intestine have a safe environment and nutrients and in return prevent the overgrowth of other bacteria.

Commensalism includes a commensal and a host. The commensal benefits and the host receives no benefit but is not harmed. The commensal shares the host's food and is therefore not dependent on the host's metabolism. This encompasses the normal flora that thrive on skin and mucous membranes of the body.

Parasitism includes a *parasite* and a *host*. The parasite benefits to the detriment of the host, such as with HIV infection where cells are invaded so the virus can propagate.

Formation of a biofilm

A biofilm is a community of a variety of bacteria and other pathogens that have banded together to form a structure held together by polysaccharide "glue." The biofilm protects the bacteria, providing increased resistance to antibiotics. Additionally, the lack of available nutrients in the biofilm forces the microorganisms to grow more slowly, making them less sensitive to antibiotics that target cells that grow fast. The stress involved in living in the biofilm causes bacteria to release acids and proteins that counteract the antibiotics and confuse the host's immune system. Biofilms have free-roaming bacteria that emerge and circulate, and these are susceptible to antibiotics, but once the drugs stop, new free-roaming bacteria emerge and the infection flares up again. Once a biofilm is established in the body, it is very difficult to treat. Many chronic infections are related to biofilms, especially with gum disease, urinary and bone infections. Invasive medical devices, such as central venous catheters and prosthesis, are common sites for biofilms.

Mechanism of phagocytosis

Phagocytosis is the mechanism by which one organism engulfs and destroys or digests another. It is a critical part of the immune response. Phagocytosis is a function of neutrophils, monocytic macrophages, and eosinophils. Macrophages may circulate or remain in fixed positions. Stages include:

- *Chemotaxis*: Neutrophils detect foreign pathogen and they and other macrophages (phagocytes) migrate toward it. Capillaries dilate to increase permeability so macrophages can attack.
- *Adherence*: The phagocyte binds to the pathogen and opsonization may take place, a process through which the pathogen is coated with antibodies and complement proteins to promote adherence.
- *Ingestion*: Pseudopods (false feet) project from the membrane of the phagocyte, surrounding the pathogen and forming a sac (phagosome) around it inside the phagocyte.
- *Digestion*: Lysosome fuses with the phagosome to create a killing structure called a phagolysosome, destroying the peptidoglycan of the cell wall, effectively killing the pathogen.
- *Excretion*: A structure called a residual body carries waste products that are discharged through the cell wall.

Bacteria-mediated vs. host-mediated pathogenesis

Infection includes the interplay and imbalance between a microorganism and the host. The virulence factor of the pathogen relates to characteristics of bacteria-mediated pathogenesis. Some bacteria produce toxins that damage cells, some have protective coatings that prevent phagocytosis by the body's defense, and others have proteins that allow them to adhere to the cells of the host, often entering the cell, resulting in cell damage or destruction. Once inside a cell, the bacteria is often safe from antibodies the host produces to fight the bacterial invasion. Host-mediated pathogenesis is related to the immune response in reaction to a bacterial infection. This response may cause as much or more damage than the bacteria. In response to some bacteria, the immune system, including lymphocytes, macrophages, and neutrophils, may release toxic factors that cause so much damage to cells that it allows the proliferation of resistant bacteria. In other cases, the lack of cellular response to some bacteria allows them to multiply rapidly.

Pathogenicity

Endotoxins

Endotoxins are lipopolysaccharide components of the outer cell wall of all Gram-negative bacteria, which are commonly found in the environment. Some of these organisms include E. Coli, Salmonella, Haemophilus, Neisseria, and Pseudomonas. All endotoxins are similar in structure and activity although there are some differences. Because endotoxins are part of the cell wall rather than excreted by it, endotoxins do the most damage after the bacterial cell is destroyed, releasing the toxin systemically. While some effects of endotoxins can benefit the host by increasing resistance to infection, other effects, such as producing fever, hypotension, leukopenia with subsequent leukocytosis, hypotension, hypothermia, and shock, can be lethal or cause severe illness. Endotoxins affect the hypothalamus by interfering with control of body temperature and cause phagocytes to release tumor necrosis factor, causing shock. Many cells and proteins in the host can bind to endotoxins causing a variety of uncontrolled host-mediated responses.

Exotoxins

Exotoxins are protein products primarily of Gram-positive bacteria, but can also be products of some Gram-negative bacteria. Organisms that produce exotoxins include *Bacillus anthraces, E. coli, Shigella dysenteriae, Clostridium tetani, Staphylococcus aureus,* and *Streptococcus pyogenes.* Exotoxins are secreted by bacteria and are more toxic than endotoxins. Different bacteria produce toxins specific to the bacteria. Some exotoxins attack specific cells, organs, or fluids within the host while others have a more general and widespread effect. Exotoxins include cytotoxins, which attack various types of cells; neurotoxins, which attack neurons in the central nervous system; and enterotoxins, which attack the cells of the intestinal mucosa. Exotoxins attach to target cells and then enter to the cell. Because they are proteins, they exert an antigenic effect and some can be neutralized by antibodies. Toxic effects for some may decrease over time as they become less toxic and convert to toxoids, maintaining antigenic properties.

Complement proteins

The complement system involves about 35 inactive proteins circulating in the blood and activating and "complementing" or assisting in destruction of pathogens. When a complement protein encounters a pathogen, a "complement cascade," a series of biochemical reactions, occur in which many protein complements coat microbes to disrupt the cell membrane, increasing susceptibility to phagocytosis. There are 3 pathways to activation:
- Classical complement cascade activates when the C1 (first protein complement) encounters an antibody attached to an antigen-antibody complex and assists the antibody. A series of complement proteins attach in a cascade, one after the other, and are able to puncture the cell membrane.
- Alternative complement cascade activates when a C3 complement protein directly attaches to a pathogen. It is useful for infections that do not involve antibodies.
- Mannan-blnding lectin (MBL) complement cascade activates when a C1q complement protein attaches to mannose and other sugars, allowing the protein to bind to many different pathogens,

Innate host defenses

Innate defenses are those that are common to healthy hosts and provide protection from pathogens. These include the following:
- *Resistance:* Species resistance includes lack of receptors for adhesins, inhospitable temperature or environment, lack of necessary nutrients, and lack of target cells for toxins. Individual resistance may be a factor of age, sex, health, medications, or many other elements.
- *natomical barriers:* Bacteria are not able to invade intact skin and the mucus and/or cilia in the mucous membranes make adherence difficult for many bacteria. Acids in the gastrointestinal tract kill many pathogens. The natural acidity of urine is not compatible with many bacteria.
- *Normal flora:* Flora compete with, inhibit, and destroy other pathogens.
- *ntimicrobial agents:* Body fluids, lymphocytes, and macrophages contain numerous proteins and protein compounds that disrupt, inhibit, or kill invading pathogens.
- *Inflammatory response: Erythema*, increased temperature, and edema aid in the functioning of the immune system.
- *Phagocytes:* Cells that can engulf and destroy pathogens are triggered by inflammation.

Antibody-mediated (humoral) immunity
Immune host defenses are more specific than innate and are directed against a specific pathogen or its byproducts. This inducible defense system develops resistance and immunity. Antibody-mediated (humoral) immunity begins when a microorganism invades a host and carries antigenic substances, which can be components of the cell wall, structures such as fimbraie, toxins or enzymes. When a macrophage encounters a pathogen, it phagocytizes and destroys it. Then the macrophage displays fragments of the antigen on its surface to activate T cells, which in turn activate B cells, which divide and form plasma cells, which release antibodies that are specific to the antigens. Antibodies are

- 37 -

immunoglobulins, of which there are 5 types. The macrophage also forms memory cells, which become part of the permanent immune system. The antibodies bind to antigens, creating what is referred to as the antigen-antibody complex, and destroying the antigen, leading to destruction of the pathogen.

Cell-mediated immunity
Cell-mediated immunity is a delayed-type hypersensitivity response (DTH) that activates cells rather than antibodies to fight pathogens. This same system is activated against transplants, causing rejection. After macrophages phagocytize antigens, proteins are encoded by major histocompatibility complex (MHC) so they can display antigenic fragments, alerting T-lymphocyte cells, which are coated with clusters of differentiation (CD), chemical molecules. The thymus releases cytotoxic T killer cells (CD8+) that can recognize the MHC carrying foreign antigen, from bacteria, viruses, tumors, or transplanted tissue. In an activation phase, T cells with the correct receptors for the pathogen divide and multiply. In the effector phase, these cytotoxic T cells release lymphotoxins that destroy the pathogenic cells. T helper (TH) cells (CD4+) secrete lymphokines that stimulate both T cells and B cells to multiply. Suppressor T-cells deactivate the immune response. Cell-mediated immunity is especially effective for viral, fungal, and protozoan infections as well as tumor cells and intracellular bacteria.

Immunoglobulins (Ig)

Functions
Immunoglobulins (Ig) are antibodies, soluble glycoproteins that serve as a defense against invasive bacteria, viruses, or parasites. The Y-shaped immunoglobulins identify foreign antigens and bind to them as part of the immune response. The ends of the Y structure contain paratroops that adhere to specific receptors, called epitopes, on antigens specific to a pathogen, signalling phagocytes to mobilize or directly destroying the pathogen. Producing immunoglobins is the primary purpose of the antibody-mediated immune response (also called the humoral immune system). Immunoglobulins attached to B cells are bound by a membrane and called B cell receptors, and serve to activate these cells. Antibodies are found in the blood and other body fluids as well as in mucoid secretions. B cells produce plasma cells that in turn secrete immunoglobulins. Ig can bind to pathogens in mucus, preventing colonization and can also bind directly to toxins. Ig neutralizes viruses, but if this is incomplete, as with HIV, the Ig increases infectivity.

Types
There are 5 different types of immunoglobulins (Ig) or antibodies (Alpha, Delta, Epsilon, Gamma, Mu), with subtypes in some cases, based on their sequences of amino acids. While these types are common to vertebrates, the base of the Y-structured immunoglobulin is specific to each animal:
- IgG has 4 subclasses and is only Ig transferred placentally. It increases opsonization, phagocytosis, and is the primary antibody-mediated immune response Ig.
- IgM has 2 subclasses and facilitates agglutination of microorganisms as well as fixing complement to lyse pathogens. IgM is part of early cell-mediated immune response.
- IgA usually does not fix complement and is found in secretions of mucous membranes.
- IgD does not fix complement and is found on B cells, but the function is unclear.
- IgE binds to basophils and mast cells before antigens, triggering release of histamine, so it is the cause of hypersensitive allergic responses. IgE also increases in helminth infection.

Normal flora

Normal flora gain access to the surface of the body by contact with the skin or the mucous membranes of the gastrointestinal, reproductive, or respiratory tracts. Normal flora are not usually found in internal organs, such as the brain or the blood. There are over 200 organisms that are part of the normal flora (mostly bacteria), which vary according to genetics, age, sex, nutrition, environment, and other factors. Many bacteria, such as *Staphylococcus aureus,* are basically pathogenic and can cause opportunistic infections. The largest numbers of flora inhabit the intestinal tract. Intestinal bacteria, such as *Escherichia coli,* have an active role in digestion and prevent colonization of other pathogens, but can also cause infection. Some flora are transient; others permanent. Flora often has tissue tropism, a preference for some types of tissues. Some have surface components that allow them to bind with host cells in order to colonize. Others build bacterial biofilms, slime glue composed primarily of capsules, or use those built by other bacteria.

The normal flora of the body are necessary and benefit the host in a number of ways.
- *Synthesis and secretion of vitamins:* Bacteria are an important source of Vitamin K and Vitamin B-12, which is secreted by enteric bacteria, such as *E. coli.*
- *Resistance to colonization:* The normal flora attaches to host cells, preventing competing bacteria from attaching and colonizing. They also compete for nutrition.
- *Inhibition or destruction of pathogens:* Bacterial flora may produce substances, such as fatty acids or bacteriocins, which destroy invading pathogens.
- *Develops tissue: In* response to normal flora, the walls of some structure, such as the cecum and some lymphatic tissue thicken and strengthen.
- *Stimulation of antibodies:* Normal flora have antigenic properties that stimulate formation of "natural" antibodies in the host. These antibodies can cross-react with the antigens of related pathogens as part of an immune response.

Specific microorganisms

Staphylococcus aureus

Staphylococcus aureus is a Gram-positive aerobic coccus that grows in clusters. *S. aureus* is commonly found on the skin, and the most common reservoir is the anterior nares. *S. aureus* is often also found in the axillae, the perineum, irritated skin, and mucous membranes. *S. aureus* attaches with surface proteins that promote colonization. *S. aureus* is not susceptible to complement protein cascade although there are antibodies that can block some receptors, preventing adhesion. However, once attached, the bacteria are coated with proteins from the host cell wall, and this shields the bacteria. *S. aureus* produces a number of exotoxins and endotoxins, including enterotoxins, toxic shock syndrome toxins, and epidermolytic toxins. *S. aureus* can become extremely virulent and can spread quickly through compromised tissue. It can spread though contact with purulent material and close contact with someone infected. *S. aureus* is a major cause of nosocomial post-operative infections, both localized and systemic, and infections from indwelling tubes and devices. There are increasingly resistant forms.

Staphylococcus aureus (MRSA)

Methicillin-resistant *Staphylococcus aureus* (MRSA) poses a serious problem. Penicillin was first introduced in 1942, and shortly thereafter, penicillin-resistant forms occurred. In 1959, methicillin was introduced to combat penicillin-resistant *S. aureus,* but within 2 years, methicillin-resistant forms were identified. Since that time, MRSA has spread throughout the world. In the United States, by 1999, MRSA infections accounted for over one-third of *Staphylococcus* infections. Many MRSA forms are resistant to multiple antibiotics and respond only to vancomycin or other investigational drugs, and there are now vancomycin-resistant forms. People who have had invasive procedures or are immunocompromised are most often infected. MRSA has numerous hospital-associated strains (HA-MRSA) that have adapted well to the hospital environment, but community-associated (CA-MRSA) forms, usually skin infections, have been isolated as well. Most HA-MRSA is caused by autoinfection in people who are already carriers with nasal carriage, frequently related to prior antibiotic use and/or prolonged hospitalization.

Streptococcus pyogenes

Group A β-hemolytic streptococci (GABHS) (*Streptococcus pyogenes*) is a Gram-positive coccus that lacks mobility and does not produce spores. It grows in pairs or chains. It is a frequent pathogen of humans, usually causing a secondary infection after a viral infection or disruption of the normal flora. Historically, GABHS has caused puerperal fever and scarlet fever, and there has been a recent increase in invasive GABHS infections, from mild pharyngitis and impetigo to severe invasive infections, including cellulites and necrotizing fascitis. GABHS infections are concerns for burn wounds as well as puerperal and neonatal infections. GABHS has numerous virulence factors that can cause a number of different diseases. It can colonize and multiply rapidly. GABHS has a hyaluronic acid capsule that contains antigens similar to those of human cells, confusing the immune system and protecting it from phagocytosis. Additionally, it produces exotoxins, such as pyrogenic toxin, which can cause toxic shock syndrome. Sequelae can include rheumatic fever and kidney disease. Most infections involve the skin or the respiratory system.

Streptococcus agalactiae

Group B β-hemolytic streptococci (GBS) (*Streptococcus agalactiae)* or Group B β-hemolytic streptococci (GBS) is a Gram-positive coccus that is part of the normal flora of the gastrointestinal system but may colonize the urogenital system of females although most infant infections are related to nosocomial rather than maternal transmission. The virulence factor of GBS relates to the protective capsule that prevents phagocytosis, thereby allowing it to colonize and multiply. GBS has been implicated in a wide range of nosocomial infections. GBS has increasingly been a cause of infections in neonatal units, causing pneumonia, meningitis, and sepsis. Meningitis can also occur in later onset, about 3-4 weeks after birth, with severe sequelae. GBS is also implicated in severe puerperal infections, but using cultures to screen women who are infected and administering antibiotics has cut infections. GBS infections may occur as wound infections after Caesarean sections, especially in women who are immunocompromised.

Streptococcus pneumoniae

Streptococcus pneumoniae is a Gram-positive elongated anaerobic coccus. It may occur singly, in pairs (most common) or in chains. It lacks motility and does not produce spores. It is part of the transient flora of the nasopharynx. *S. pneumoniae* is encased in a polysaccharide capsule that prevents phagocytosis. The cell wall activates the alternative complement cascade (among others), causing an inflammatory reaction and as the *S.pneumoniae* it destroyed, it releases pneumolysin and other cytotoxins that increase inflammation, kill cells, and can cause septic shock. The cell wall is composed of 6 layers of peptidoglycan and contains choline that allows it to adhere to cells with choline-binding receptors, including almost all human cells. *S. pneumoniae* has a transformation system that allows it to easily mutate and develop resistance to antibiotics. It is the most common cause lobar pneumonia in adults, and there have been frequent outbreaks in nursing homes. Immunization is the primary method of prevention.

Enterococci

Enterococci are Gram-positive facultative anaerobic (preferring oxygen but able to survive without it) cocci that usually occur in pairs. Only a few of the 21 species cause human infections. *Enterococci* are part of the normal flora of the gastrointestinal tract, which is the reservoir for most nosocomial infections, but they can also be found on skin, wounds, and chronic decubitus ulcers. They were formerly classified as *Streptococci* and look similar. *E. faecalis* causes 60-90% of infections and *E. feacium* causes 5-16%, but *E. feacium* is of increasing concern because it has developed vancomycin resistant strains. *Enterococci* are difficult to treat because they are intrinsically resistant to numerous antibiotics, including penicillins and cephalosporins. Additionally, they have acquired resistance to many others, including tetracyclines and vancomycin. Infections include urinary infections, bacteremia, endocarditis as well as infections in wounds and the abdominal and pelvic areas. Person-to-person transmission is common in nosocomial infections.

Vancomycin resistant *enterococci* (VRE) and multi-drug resistant *enterococci* (MDRE)

Vancomycin resistant *enterococci* (VRE) and multi-drug resistant *enterococci* (MDRE) have become severe cause for concern. VRE was first identified in the United States in 1989, but by 2004 it was the cause of one-third of all hospital-acquired infections in intensive care units, related to the use of vancomycin. There are several phenotypes, but 2 types are most common in the United States: VanA (resistant to vancomycin and teicoplanin) and Van B (resistant to just van VRE infections are treatable by other antibiotics, but MDRE infections are increasingly resistant to 2 or more antibiotics, including vancomycin. Restriction of vancomycin use alone has not proven successful in controlling development of VRE or MDRE because other antibiotics, such as clindamycin, cephalosporin, aztreonam, ciprofloxacin, aminoglycoside, and metronidazole are implicated. Prior antibiotic use is present in almost all patients with MDRE. Other risk factors include prolonged hospitalization and intraabdominal surgery.

Enterobacteriaceae

Enterobacteriaceae are facultative anaerobic Gram-negative bacilli that are part of the natural flora of the gastrointestinal tract. They are also commonly found in the soil, water, and plants. Most have flagella for motility, and they don't produce spores. *Enterobacteriaceae* comprise numerous genera, including *Escherichia coli, Shigella, Salmonella, Klebsiella, Enterobacter, Proteus,* and *Yersinia.* Virulence varies according to the ability of the organism to metabolize lactose. Those that do not are usually pathogenic. Adherence factors also impact virulence as some genera and species have more effective adhesins than others. *Enterobacteriaceae* produce toxins that can be extremely dangerous. *Enterobacteriaceae* cause less than a third of nosocomial infections, a decreasing number. However, they cause about half of the urinary tract infections and a quarter of the postoperative infections, and increasing resistance to antibiotics increases the risk of sepsis, diarrhea, and meningitis. Many species are able to cause symptoms that are similar, so identifying the pathogen is important.

Escherichia coli of the family *Enterobacteriaceae*

Escherichia coli, a facultative anaerobic Gram-negative bacillus, is part of the normal flora of the intestines. There are hundreds of serotypes of *E.coli,* based on O, H, and K antigens. *E.coli* serves a necessary role in digestion and production of Vitamin K and B-complex vitamins as well as suppressing growth of harmful bacteria that may invade the intestines; however, it is also the biggest cause of urinary infections and some strains, such as O157:H7 are extremely virulent, causing severe diarrhea, hemolytic uremia, and death. There are 5 classes of diarrhea-producing *E. coli.. E.coli* produces both endotoxins and exotoxins that causes diarrhea, and since death of the organism releases toxins, antibiotic treatment can make some infections and symptoms worse. As a nosocomial infection, *E.coli* primarily causes urinary tract infections (especially related to catheters), diarrhea, and neonatal meningitis but it can also lead to pneumonia, and bacteremia (usually secondary to urinary infection). Endotoxins can cause intravascular coagulation and death.

Pseudomonas aeruginosa

Pseudomonas aeruginosa is a Gram-negative aerobic bacillus that is ubiquitous in soil and water, favoring moist conditions. It can grow in the absence of oxygen if nitrate is available. P. aeruginosa has fimbriae that facilitate adherence to epithelial cells in the respiratory tract. P. aeruginosa is encapsulated, providing protection from antibodies, and produces toxins, enzymes, cytotoxins, and hemolysins that resist phagocytosis and destroy cells of the host. P. aeruginosa is an opportunistic infection, invading compromised tissue. It can cause severe infections of virtually all systems and is especially dangerous for those with severe burns or with immunosuppression. Additionally, P.

aeruginosa is resistant to many common antibiotics and some strains have proven resistant to all antimicrobials. Because P. aeruginosa has a high virulence factor, it can easily invade the bloodstream, causing bacteremia, which carries a 40% mortality rate. Bacteremia may also result from contaminated liquids and equipment, such as endoscopes.

Mycobacterium tuberculosis

Mycobacterium tuberculosis is a non-motile obligate aerobic bacillus that forms chains, which are associated with a toxic surface component called cord factor. *M. tuberculosis* is neither Gram-negative nor positive. As an extracellular agent, it needs oxygen, so it is attracted to the upper respiratory tract. It is also a facultative intracellular invader, allowing it to evade the immune system. Humans serve as the reservoir for this pathogen. The virulence is increased because of a unique cell wall composed of peptidoglycan but also complex lipids that provide antibiotic resistance and include acids that protect the cell, cord factor that is toxic to host cells, and Wax-D, which protects the cell envelope. The host immune system attempts to control the spread of *M. tuberculosis* by walling it off with macrophages, causing a positive skin reaction (cell-mediated immune response) but no infection. Resistant strains are an increasing cause of concern. Nosocomial outbreaks have occurred, often related to failure to identify an infected source.

Multi-drug resistant tuberculosis (MDR-TB) is resistant to at least 2 commonly used first-line drugs, isoniazid (INH) and rifampin, while extensively drug resistant tuberculosis (XDR-TB) is also resistant to all fluoroquinolones and at least one of the three second-line drugs: amikacin, kanamycin, or capreomycin.

XDR-TB emerged as a worldwide concern in 2005. In the United States, it is at present most commonly found in foreign born patients but also occurs in immunocompromised patients. Active TB requires treatment for extended periods of time, usually 18-24 months, with multiple drugs. Since the 1980s there has been increased need to use second-line drugs to combat infection. There are two primary causes for the increased resistance:
- Failure to complete a course of treatment
- Mismanaged treatment, including incorrect medication, dosage, or duration of therapy.

People who have had previous TB are at increased risk and should be monitored carefully. Drug resistant TB increasingly poses a risk for patients and staff in healthcare facilities.

The infection control plan should include provisions for referring patients and/or staff with tuberculosis for directly-observed therapy (DOT) when indicated. DOT requires that a healthcare worker monitor every dose of an individual's anti-tuberculosis medication, ensuring that all medications are taken and the entire course of treatment is completed. Drug protocol may be changed to 2-3 times weekly rather than daily to facilitate DOT. Regulations about DOT vary from state to state. DOT is frequently used in these circumstances:
- Sputum cultures are positive for acid-fast bacilli.
- There is concurrent treatment with antiretroviral (HIV) drugs or methadone (for addiction).
- Infection is MDR-TB or XDR-TB.
- Co-morbidity with psychiatric disease or cognitive impairment exists.
- Patient is homeless and lacks adequate facilities.
- Patient has demonstrated lack of reliability in treatment.

When patients are discharged from the hospital, plans must include continuation of DOT through the use of home health agencies or having the patient return to a clinic for administration of drugs.

Clostridium difficile

Clostridium difficile is an anaerobic Gram-positive bacillus that produces endospores. It is commonly found in healthcare facilities. Normal intestinal flora provide resistance to *C. difficile,* but if the flora is disrupted by antibiotic use (or sometimes chemotherapeutic agents) and the host is an asymptomatic carrier or has acquired the infection during or after treatment, then *C. difficile* can begin to overgrow. *C. difficile* produces a lethal cytotoxin (Toxin B) and an endotoxin with cytotoxic action (Toxin A) that causes fluid to accumulate in the colon and severe damage to mucous membranes. *C. difficile* causes more nosocomial diarrhea cases than any other microorganism. All antibiotics can cause *C. difficile* infections but Clindamycin and cephalosporins are most-frequently implicated. Symptoms vary widely, from mild diarrhea to lethal sepsis. It can cause diarrhea, colitis, and pseudomembranous colitis, and megacolon. Infection may not be obvious for weeks after completion of antibiotics.

Legionella

Legionella is a Gram-negative obligate aerobic bacillus that is motile. *Legionella* is comprised of 48 species, but *L. pneumophila* causes 90% of infections, most often in those who are immunocompromised. *Legionella* is an intracellular pathogenic agent that replicates within monocytic phagocytes (depending on the availability of iron) and alveolar macrophages. Both antibody-mediated (which can result in long-term resistance) and cell-mediated immunity responses occur to combat infection. *Legionella* colonizes water distribution systems because it can survive chlorine treatment. It grows well in hot water tanks. Air-conditioning systems, despite wide belief, have not been implicated in the spread of infection. Nosocomial infections correlate with use of ventilators, intubation, and naso-gastric tubes. Using tap water instead of sterile water to cleanse equipment can lead to infection. The most common infections are Pontiac fever, which is flu-like, and pneumonia, which can lead to dissemination of the pathogen throughout the body, causing multi-organ failure.

Candida

Candida is a yeast fungal pathogen. C. albicans is the most common, but non-C. albicans pathogenic forms, some resistant to antifungal medications, have caused nosocomial outbreaks. Humans and animals are the reservoirs for Candida, and C. albicans is part of the normal flora of mucous membranes and can cause superficial infections, such as thrush and vaginitis. Candida species can adhere to multiple host tissues, but an intact cell-mediated immune system can limit infection, but if this immune system is defective (as with AIDS) Candida can overgrow and lead to mucocutaneous or cutaneous lesions and sepsis. Candida multiplies in a bioform structure that provides protection from antifungals. Intact skin is an effective barrier, but lesions, burns, and intravascular tubes can allow invasion. Normal intestinal flora also suppress Candida, but disruption caused by antimicrobials allows infection. C. tropicalis can cause invasive candidiasis, particularly in leukemia patients. C. parapsilosis is an environmental contaminant and can be transferred on the hands and causes infections of the bloodstream.

Aspergillus spp

Aspergillus spp. are filamentous (having long threads) fungi, which increasingly cause nosocomial infections. They are ubiquitous in the environment and are aerobic, grow as molds, and produce spores that become airborne and can invade the respiratory tract. There are about 180 species, but about 20 are human pathogens. Most healthy people are resistant to *Aspergillus,* but it can invade almost all organs, although rarely infecting the blood. Invasive infections occur in those who are immunocompromised, such as those having transplants or receiving chemotherapy. Mortality rates are as high as 90% for invasive infections and treatment often involves surgical debridement as well as medical treatment. Mold remediation, high efficiency particulate air (HEPA) filtration and laminar airflow rooms have been used to avoid infection, and antifungal prophylaxis may also be indicated. *A. fumigatus* and *flavus* cause most invasive infections. *A. fumigatus* and *clavatus* activate the antigen-antibody immune response, causing a hypersensitivity reaction.

Influenza viruses A & B

Influenza A is more virulent and common than influenza B, but both have been linked to epidemics and pose threats to those hospitalized, especially young or elderly. Influenza A is an avian virus that has migrated to humans while Influenza B only affects humans, which are reservoirs for both. Influenza viruses are round or filamentous and have an RNA (single-strand) genome, which is in 8 segments inside a protein envelope. The segmented genome allows for new strains to develop easily and quickly, making vaccines short-lived. The virus binds to the host cell, allowing entry of the RNA into the host. The genes are copied and the host cell begins producing viral particles. Influenza viruses stimulate the antibody-mediated immune response. Influenza infections usually present as fever, chills, myalgia, and cough but can progress to viral pneumonia and secondary bacterial pneumonia. Transmission is by droplet particles directly to mucous membranes or by infected hands making contact with mucous membranes.

Varicella-zoster virus

Varicella-zoster virus (Human herpes virus 3) in the herpesvirus family causes both chicken pox, and herpes zoster (shingles). The varicella-zoster virus contains double-strands of DNA and has a protective envelope. Once it gains entry to a host from airborne droplets, it begins to replicate. A rash, initially red that becomes vesicular, appears about 2 weeks after initial infection with the infection running its course in 10-21 days. While most chickenpox infections are mild, they can result in viral encephalitis or pneumonia, especially in those who are immunocompromised. After infection, the host's antibody-mediated immune response confers immunity to chicken pox: however, the virus remains dormant in the dorsal root ganglia or the cranial nerve ganglia and can become reactivated. Reactivation results in herpes zoster, involving severe pain along the involved nerve and a vesicular rash, usually around the trunk or the head. Pain can persist for weeks or months. Herpes zoster is spread by direct contact with vesicles, causing chickenpox in those who are not immune.

Herpes simplex virus I and II

Herpes simplex virus I causes herpetic lesions primarily on the lips and face, a "cold sore," and is spread directly by contact with infected lesions, often through kissing or oral sex. Herpes simplex virus II causes lesions primarily in the urogenital area and is spread by sexual contact. Both types can occur in either area or on other areas of the body. Between infections, both viruses remain in a latent state and can be reactivated. Herpes I usually migrates to the trigeminal root ganglia while Herpes II remains dormant in the sacral plexus. The antibody-mediated immune response controls latency, during which the virus replicates much more slowly, but can reactivate during illness, fever, or times of stress. When the immune system is compromised, the virus can reactivate and spread out of control causing severe, large, painful lesions and may result in encephalitis, pneumonia esophagitis, ocular disease, and proctitis. Patients and staff with active lesions can spread herpes, resulting in nosocomial outbreaks in infants and adults.

Cytomegalovirus

Cytomegalovirus (CMV) in the herpes virus family and contains DNA in its genome. The cell envelope is formed from the cell membranes of budding virions. Outside of the host, the virus is easily destroyed by disinfectants. CMV infections are ubiquitous in humans and are usually asymptomatic but may cause a mononucleosis-type illness in some. CMV is much more serious in those who are immunocompromised as it can invade and replicate in any organ in the body and has been implicated in transplant rejection. People may develop pneumonia, liver infection, and anemia. CMV also poses a threat to pregnant women and to the fetus of a newly-infected mother. CMV retinitis is a serious complication of HIV infection, increasing as the CD4 count decreases. CMV can be transmitted placentally, in body fluids, and on the hands, a common cause of nosocomial transmission; therefore, handwashing procedures are extremely important to prevent nosocomial transmission and infection.

Hepatitis A virus (HAV)

Hepatitis A virus (HAV) is an RNA picornavirus that replicates in the liver, is secreted into the gallbladder and enters the intestines. The virus triggers an antibody-mediated immune response with IgM that confers immunity, so reinfection and chronic infection does not occur. HAV infection is often asymptomatic in children, but adults may develop jaundice, general malaise, pain in the abdomen, nausea, and diarrhea. The virus is transmitted by the oral-fecal route through contamination with fecal material, often on the hands or through sexual contact. On rare occasions, HAV has been transmitted in blood transfusions. . Because infants are usually asymptomatic, infection with HAV may not be suspected in neonatal units. Nosocomial infections have occurred when there has been a break in infection control and HAV from infected stool of infants or adults with diarrhea was transmitted on the hands of staff. Vaccine is available but not routinely administered.

Hepatis B virus (HBV)

Hepatitis B virus (HBV) is a DNA of the family *Hepadnaviridae* and is transmitted through contact with blood either directly or through sexual contact or sharing needles. The DNA genome enters the host cell nucleus, copies, and replicates. The cell-mediated immune response that destroys the virus also causes damage to hepatic cells, resulting in acute hepatitis. Chronic infection occurs in 90% of infants and 6% of those over 5 years old, with 15-25% of those with chronic infection developing liver cancer. The virus can remain stable in the environment for a week. Outbreaks in healthcare facilities have occurred because of contaminated blood-sampling and hemodialysis equipment as well as from the use of multi-dose vials. Using single-dose vials and disposable equipment as well as proper handwashing techniques are important for prevention of nosocomial infections. Vaccine is available and advised for healthcare workers who may come in contact with blood. . Children are now routinely vaccinated for HBV.

Hepatitis C virus (HCV)

Hepatitis C virus (HCV) is a single-strand RNA *Flaviviridae* virus that binds to receptors on hepatic cells and enters to begin replicating. HCV readily mutates, which helps it to evade the host's immune response. There are 6 genotypes and several subtypes of HCV with some types more virulent and resistive to treatment than others. There is no vaccine. HCV is transmitted directly through blood or items, such as shared needles, contaminated with blood. It can be spread by sexual contact. Prior to 1992, the blood supply was contaminated with HCV as was clotting factors made before 1987. HCV causes an acute infection (first 6 months), but 55-85% develop chronic infection with 70% of those developing chronic liver disease. HCV is the primary reasons for liver transplants. Nosocomial infections are similar to HBV and related to contaminated blood sampling equipment, multidose vials, improperly sterilized equipment, and breakdown in infection control methods.

Human immunodeficiency virus (HIV)

Human immunodeficiency virus (HIV) is a slow-acting retrovirus of the genus lentivirus. HIV binds with cells that have CD4 receptors, primarily CD4+ T cells and other cells of the immune system, enters the cells and begins replicating. Host cells are destroyed in a number of ways:

- *Disruption of cell wall or cellular function* may be caused after large numbers of replicated viral cells bud through the cell membrane or build up inside the cell.
- *Formation of syncytia* occurs when cells infected with HIV fuse with nearby cells creating giant cells, thus allowing HIV to spread from one cell to many.
- *poptosis,* or cell death, occurs when HIV sends a signal to uninfected cells, causing them to self-destruct.
- *inding to cell surface* of uninfected cell by HIV gives the appearance that the cell is infected, causing it to be targeted by killer T cells as part of the immune response.

HIV is spread through blood or other bodily fluids and blood-contaminated equipment.

Scabies

Scabies is caused by a microscopic mite, *Sarcoptes scabiei hominis,* which tunnel under the outer layer of skin, raising small lines a few millimeters long. Mites prefer warm areas, such as between the fingers and in skin folds, but can infest any area of the body. As the mites burrow, they cause intense itching and subsequent scratching can result in secondary infections. Scabies is spread very easily through person-to-person contact and has become a problem in nursing homes and extended care facilities where staff spread the infection from one patient to another. Incubation time is 6-8 weeks and itching usually begins in about 30 days, so people may be unaware they are transmitting scabies. Most infestations involve only about a dozen mites, but a severe form of scabies infection, Norwegian or crusted scabies, can occur in the elderly or those who are immunocompromised. In this case, lesions can contain thousands of mites, making this type highly contagious.

Chagas disease

Chagas disease, caused by the protozoan parasite *Trypanosoma cruzi,* is endemic to much of Mexico, Central, and South America, and is transmitted when a triatomine insect bites the skin and deposits contaminated feces in the wound. The parasite invades organs and is transmitted through blood and organ donations. Chagas is an emerging disease in the United States where a large Latin American immigrant population has brought between 100,000 to 625,000 cases. Chagas has 3 stages, acute with either no or flu-like symptoms for most people, an intermediate stage that is asymptomatic and a chronic stage that occurs about 30 years after infection, presenting with severe cardiomyopathy and digestive problems. People are often unaware that they are infected but pose a danger to the blood supply. Treatment is often ineffective after the acute stage. Most blood banks have begun testing for Chagas disease. Only universal precautions should be necessary for Chagas disease.

Pathogenesis terms

Adherence: Adherence is using a mechanism to attach a microorganism to a host. Adherence requires an adhesin in the microorganism and a receptor in the host.
Antitoxin: Antitoxin is an antibody that has the ability to bind to an exotoxin and neutralize it.
Cytotoxin: Cytotoxin is a type of exotoxin that disrupts and destroys the cells of host. There are numerous varieties.
Endotoxin: Endotoxin is a toxin made of protein, lipid, and polysaccharides. It develops in the outer cell wall of Gram-negative bacteria and is extremely toxic, sometimes causing sepsis and death.
Enterotoxin: Enterotoxin (cytoenterotoxin) is a type of cytotoxin that targets the cells of the intestinal mucosa. Most types form spores in cell membranes, killing the cell.
Exotoxin: Exotoxin is a protein or enzyme that is produced by bacteria and released from the cell, usually into the blood stream, where it disrupts metabolism of cells and destroys them. Some are extremely toxic.
Neurotoxin: Neurotoxin is a type of cytotoxin that specifically targets neurons in the central nervous system, leading to paralysis.
ID50: ID50/ED 50 (infectious/ effective dose 50%) is the number of microorganisms that is needed to cause infection in half of the hosts that have been exposed.
LD50: LD50 (lethal dose 50%) is the number of microorganism that is needed to cause death in half of the hosts that have been exposed.
Pathogenicity: Pathogenicity is the ability of an organism to cause disease.
Toxemia: Toxemia is the condition in which there are toxins in the blood system.
Toxicity: Toxicity is the degree of virulence related to a toxin.
Toxigenicity: Toxigenicity is the ability of a microorganism to produce toxins that cause illness or death.

Toxin: Toxin is a chemical substance, usually a protein, produced by one organism that is poisonous to another.

Toxoid: Toxoid is an exotoxin that has been chemically inactivated so that it can confer immunity but not disease.

Classification of microorganisms

Viruses

Viruses (virions) are sub-microscopic and generally considered non-living because they lack cell structures. Viruses consist of nucleic acid, single or double-strand DNA and/or RNA (the genome), encapsulated in a protein coating called a capsid. Some have a lipid envelope about the capsid with glycoprotein spikes. The purpose of viruses is to reproduce, but they require a host cell with a protein receptor to which a virus must bind to penetrate the cell membrane. The viral genome carries encoding that allows it to use the cell to replicate in a *lytic* or *lysogenic* cycle. In the lytic cycle, the virus forces the cell to manufacture proteins and new genomes. After new viral particles form, the cell ruptures, releasing the viruses. In a lysogenic cycle, the virus integrates the DNA of the host and as the cell replicates, the virus replicates with it. The virus remains dormant until it activates and begins a lytic cycle. Viruses that infect bacteria are *bacteriophages* (or *phages).*

Retroviruses
Retroviruses are a sub-category of viruses. Retroviruses must have 3 characteristics: a genome that contains ribonucleic acid (RNA), the enzyme reverse transcriptase, and a protein body surrounding by a protein envelope. While some viruses contain DNA, retroviruses do not. After the virus enters the cell of a host, the reverse transcriptase uses the RNA genome to make DNA copies of the genome. Since genetic information was previously believed to transmit from DNA to RNA, this process was considered backward "retro," thus the name retrovirus. After the DNA copy is made, it invades one of the host cell's chromosomes and becomes part of the genetic makeup of the cell. To date, two retroviruses are known to infect human hosts: HTLV-1, which causes adult T-cell leukemia and HIV (human immunodeficiency virus). By invading T-helper lymphocyte cells, HIV attacks and disrupts the immune system that should detect and destroy pathogens.

Corona viruses
Corona viruses are relatively large RNA viruses that appear to have a crown or halo about them when viewed microscopically. They were first identified in chickens in 1937. A number of different corona viruses have been identified as pathogens of animals, such as dogs, and by 2005, 5 different human corona viruses had been identified, but more may exist. Corona viruses are inhaled or ingested by oral-fecal route into the respiratory system where they cause both upper and lower respiratory infection or into the gastrointestinal system where they cause gastroenteritis. They are believed to be responsible for 10-30% of viruses that cause the "common cold"; however, they are implicated in more serious infections, such as Severe Acute Respiratory Syndrome (SARS). Corona viruses replicate in cytoplasm after they enter into the host cell by endocytosis and membrane fusion. Reinfections can occur, suggesting that there are a number of different serotypes.

Satellite viruses and prions
Satellite viruses are essentially parasitic viruses that coinfect with a *helper* virus, which allows the satellite to use helper protein to replicate along with the helper virus. Hepatitis B may have a coinfection with the satellite virus, Hepatitis Delta, increasing the virulence of the infection.

Prions (derived from "Proteinaceous" and "infection) are proteins that cause infection, casting some doubt on the long held belief that DNA and RNA were the molecules required for life. Originally described as a "slow virus," a prion is not bacterial, viral, or fungal, and it can cause genetic, infectious, or sporadic disorders. In all of these disorders, prion proteins (PrP) are modified. In fact, the concept of prions is so bizarre that some researchers insist it doesn't exist. Prions are implicated in animal (mad cow disease) and human diseases in which the prions invade and destroy brain cells, transmissible spongiform encecephalopathies (Creutzfeldt-Jakob disease).

Bacteria

Bacteria are critical for human survival and most are benign, but some are pathogenic, leading to infection. Bacteria are ubiquitous, with about 10 times as many bacteria in the human body as there are human cells. Bacteria have simple prokaryote structures, with no membrane-encased nucleus or organelles but a tangle of looped DNA called a nucleoid. Bacteria also have plasmids, which are double strands of DNA outside of the nucleoid that allow for transmission from cell to cell or by attaching to viruses. Essentially, bacteria are able to trade genes, making them very adaptable. The cell membrane of most bacteria, except the Mollicutes (mycoplasmas), is surrounded by a cell wall, the composition of which varies. It's the composition of this cell wall that determines the Gram-staining, either negative or positive. Bacteria have 4 different shapes:
- Round (cocci): These occur in chains or in clusters.
- Rod-shaped (bacilli): These occur singly, doubly, or in filaments.
- Spiral (spirillum).
- Incomplete spirals (*Vibrios*)

Characteristics
Bacteria are often differentiated according to enzymes and genes that are sub-microscopic. Characteristics may vary:
- *Motility:* Some lack motility and others move by means of flagella or through creeping movements.
- *Environment:* Some bacteria are aerobic, requiring oxygen; others are anaerobic. Obligate anaerobes cannot survive in the presence of oxygen. Many are facultative anaerobes and prefer anaerobic conditions but can survive in either environment. Still other bacteria depend on other substances for survival, including sulfate, nitrite, and carbon dioxide.
- *Reproduction:* Bacteria reproduce through fission or by the production of spores. Some bacteria, primarily those found in water, soil, and human intestines, produce endospores, which seem to be able to survive indefinitely and are resistant to heat, light, solvents, and chemicals. Spores are usually activated by heat or age.
- *Nutrition:* Bacteria acquire food in different ways. Some (autotrophics) bacteria are able to manufacture their own food. Others (heterotrophics) gain nutrition from other organisms. Heterotrophics include those that cause disease.

Clinical classification
Clinical classification of bacteria takes into account those characteristics that are helpful in identifying infectious processes:
- *Gram-positive or Gram-negative status: Most* bacteria are Gram-negative stains (red) or Gram-positive (purple) although a few cannot be identified by staining. While Gram stain isn't used to identify bacteria, it's frequently referred to clinically.
- *Taxonomic status:* Taxonomy is based on the genera and species of a bacterium, but this can be confusing because some names have changed or two names are used. Genome sequencing should standardize identification.

- *Anaerobic/aerobic status:* Some bacteria are strictly anaerobic, but very few are strictly aerobic. Those that have flexibility and can grow in either aerobic or anaerobic conditions are called *facultative.*
- *Usual environment:* Bacteria are classified according to where they usually reside as flora or where they usually cause infection.
- *Virulence factor:* Bacteria vary widely in virulence. Some are actively invasive but others only cause opportunistic infections.

Colonization

In order to colonize a host, bacteria must first attach, through a mechanism called adherence. Attachment must be able to counter washing or the flow of mucous that protects mucous membranes. This requires an adhesin on the surface of the pathogen to interact with a receptor, usually a carbohydrate or peptide, on the surface of the host cell. Ligands (surface molecules), fimbriae (filaments of proteins), and pili (shorter filaments) may all serve as adhesins. Fimbriae and pili protrude from the surface of the bacteria, increasing the ability to adhere. Some components of bacterial cell walls, such as lipopolysaccharide, teichoic and lipoteichoic acids, may also be adhesins. Adherence has some degree of specificity: bacteria may exhibit a preference for one type of cell or tissue, or one type of species. Adherence may be temporary (reversible) or permanent. Bacteria may exhibit different adhesins or different types of fimbriae.

Invasin

Bacteria produce extracellular invasins, which are proteins (enzymes) that deter the host's defense system and damage cells in order to promote colonization. Invasins are in some ways similar to exotoxins but are usually less toxic and function locally rather than at a distance from the site of invasion. Some enzymes, spreading factors, affect tissue and intercellular spaces to facilitate colonization and spread.

- Hyaluronidase attacks connective tissue and is produced by *Streptococci, Staphylococci,* and *Clostridia.*
- Collagenase interferes with collagen in muscles. It is produced by *Clostridia.*
- *Neuramidase* breaks down intercellular elements of intestinal mucosa and is produced by intestinal pathogens, such as *Shigella dysenteriae.*
- *Streptokinase* (produced by *Streptococci)* and *Staphylokinase* (produced by *Staphylococcus)* promotes destruction of fibrin and prevents the blood from clotting.

Other enzymes attack the host's cell walls, leading to destruction of the cell. Some enzymes attack red cells (hemolysins) and others phagocytes (leukocidins).

Gram-negative bacteria

The cell walls of Gram-negative bacteria are characterized by red staining. The cell wall is thinner than that of Gram-positive bacteria; however, there are two separate layers to the wall: a thin inner layer of peptidoglycan (carbohydrate polymers bound by proteins), an intervening periplasmic space, and the outer membranous layer (the lipopolysaccharide layer), which produces endotoxins, making Gram-negative bacteria extremely pathogenic. A component of the outer layer is called the S-layer; it aids in adherence and protection from pathogens. The outer layer serves to protect Gram-negative organisms from antibiotics or detergents that would disrupt the inner peptidoglycan layer and provides resistance to penicillin and other compounds. Ampicillin is able to penetrate the exterior wall although many bacteria have become resistant. Common Gram-negative cocci (round) bacteria include

- *Neisseria gonorrhoeae*
- *Neisseria meningitides*

- *Moraxella catarrhalis*

Common Gram-negative bacilli (rods) include:
- *Hemophilus influenzae*
- *Legionella pneumophila*
- *Pseudomonas aeruginosa*
- *Escherichia coli*
- *Helicobacter pylori*
- *Salmonella enteritidis and typhi*

Gram-positive bacteria

Gram-positive bacteria are characterized by purple staining; the cell walls tend to be thicker than those of Gram-negative bacteria. About 90% of the cell wall of Gram-positive bacteria is made of peptidoglycan (carbohydrate polymers bound by proteins). The number of peptidoglycan layers varies, but can be more than 20, making a thick-walled cell. An S-layer is attached to the peptidoglycan layer to protect the cell and aid in adherence. Gram-positive organisms tend to be easier to kill than Gram-negative because they lack the outer wall of Gram-negative organisms, and they are more sensitive to penicillin although there are resistant strains. Peptidoglycan does not occur naturally in the human body, so it is easily recognized by the immune system as an invading organism.

Common Gram-positive cocci bacteria include:
- *Streptococcus pneumoniae*
- *Staphylococcus aureus*
- *Enterococcus*

Common Gram-positive bacilli bacteria include:
- *Corynbacterium diphtheriae*
- *Listeria monocytogenes*
- *Bacillus anthracis.*

Fungi

Fungi were originally classified as plants, but they do not produce their own food through photosynthesis and must, like animals, get the food from another source. Fungi vary widely, from one-celled microorganisms to multi-celled chains that are miles long. Fungi are used to make antibiotics, but they can also cause infection and disease. Two common classifications of fungi are molds (including mushrooms) and yeast. Fungi are not motile, but some produce spores, which can be inhaled. Some, such as the yeast *Candida albicans*, are part of the normal flora of the skin but can overgrow in an opportunistic infection. As microorganisms, fungal infections can invade the sinuses, the mouth, the respiratory system, and the vagina. Antibiotics may affect the balance between bacteria and yeast, causing infection. Fungal infections include histoplasmosis, blastomycosis, and coccidioidomycosis. Fungal infections, such as *Pneumocystis jiroveci (*formerly *carinii)* pose a serious problem for the immunocompromised. Antifungal drugs are available, but systemic fungal infections are difficult to treat.

Protozoa

Protozoa are single-cell microorganisms with a nucleus that live primarily off of bacteria. They share similarities to animals, but (except for Myxozoa) they are not, but they are also not plants. Many protozoa are free living and are ubiquitous in soil and water. They are often divided according to their method of locomotion: flagellates, amoeboids, sporozoans, and ciliates. Some protozoa are able to form protective cysts, which can survive outside the host, sometimes for long periods, before transmission to another host. Protozoa are parasites to humans and cause a wide range of infections. Enteric protozoa, such as *Giardia intestinalis* and *Entamoeba histolytica,* can cause severe diarrhea. Other diseases caused by protozoa include malaria, Chagas disease, babesiosis, toxoplasmosis, trichomonas infection, and amoebic dysentery. Protozoa take a huge toll of life, especially in developing countries, but some diseases, such as Chagas disease, or becoming more common in the United States as people emigrate from endemic areas of Latin America.

Surveillance and Epidemiologic Investigation

Design of Surveillance Systems

National Nosocomial Infections Surveillance (NNIS) system

In 1970, the National Centers for Infectious Diseases of the U.S. Centers for Disease Control and Prevention (CDC) established the National Nosocomial Infections Surveillance (NNIS) system. The purpose was to help encourage hospitals to report and track nosocomial infections and to use standardized methods to collect and analyze data and to create a national database. About 300 hospitals, whose identify remains confidential, reported data using "surveillance components" and protocols that had been standardized and used CDC definitions. Surveillance components included:
- Adult and pediatric Intensive Care Units (ICUs).
- High-risk nurseries (HRNs).
- Surgical patients
- Antimicrobial use and resistance

All ICU and HRN patients were surveyed, but hospitals chose from a list of surgical procedures those that they wanted to monitor for surgical patients as the numbers of procedures done at different hospitals can vary widely. Statistics regarding infections were compiled and issued in reports about every 3 years.

National Healthcare Safety Network

The National Healthcare Safety Network (NHSN) integrates and replaces 3 separate programs: National Nosocomial Infections Surveillance (NNIS), Dialysis Surveillance Network (DSN), and National Surveillance System for Health Care Workers (NaSH). All healthcare facilities, such as hospitals and dialysis centers, can participate in the Internet-based program that allows for reporting and sharing data. Those who apply to become members must agree to utilize CDC definitions, follow strict protocols, and submit data every 6 months. Anonymity of the institutions is protected. The program streamlines reporting of data and provides comparative data from across the United States. The system can identify sentinel or unusual events and notify appropriate participating agencies. There are 3 components to NHSN: patient safety, healthcare worker safety, and research and development. Extensive data analysis features are part of the program. Reports of nosocomial, or hospital-acquired, infections that were previously issued by NNIS are now issued by NHSN.

Developing a Surveillance System Plan

Identifying nosocomial infections
Nosocomial infection is defined by National Nosocomial Infections Surveillance (NNIS) as a hospital-acquired infection, either localized or systemic, caused by a pathogen or toxin that was not present (or incubating) in the patient at the time he/she entered the hospital. In some cases, infection may be obvious within the first 24-48 hours, but other infections may not be obvious until after discharge from the hospital because incubation times and resistance varies. An infection that occurs after discharge but is hospital-acquired is nosocomial. Identifying a nosocomial infection should result from analysis of laboratory findings as well as clinical symptoms.

A diagnosis of infection by an attending physical or surgeon is also considered acceptable identification. Placentally-transferred infections are not considered nosocomial, but perinatal infections are, even if acquired from the mother during delivery. Colonization that is not causing an inflammatory response or evidence of infection is not considered nosocomial for reporting purposes.

Purpose of surveillance plans
The purpose of a surveillance plan should be clearly outlined and may be multifaceted, including the following elements:
- *Decreasing rates of infection:* The primarily purpose of a surveillance plan is to identify a means to decrease nosocomial infections.
- *Evaluating infection control measures:* Surveillance can evaluate effectiveness of infection control measures.
- *Establishing endemic threshold rates:* Establishing threshold rates can help to enact control measures to reduce rates.
- *Identifying outbreaks:* About 5-10% of infections occur in outbreaks, and comparing data with established endemic threshold rates can help to identify these outbreaks if analysis is done in a regular and timely manner.
- *Achieving staff compliance:* Objective evidence may convince staff to cooperate with infection control measures.
- *Meeting accreditation standards:* Some accreditation agencies require reports of infection rates.
- *Providing defense for malpractice suits:* Providing evidence that a facility is proactive in combating infections can decrease liability.
- *Comparing infection rates with other facilities:* Comparing data helps focus attention and resources.

Surveillance plan steps
The steps to surveillance programs may vary to some degree, but usually contain the following elements:
- *Establishment of parameters/design* of the survey by determining what will be surveyed, when, and how with clear definitions of events guides the process.
- *Data collection* should be done consistently, efficiently, and accurately whether by hand or automated system. Sources may include laboratory reports, medical records of targeted patients, interviews, and autopsy reports.
- *Data summary* must be done so that information is accessible and available for further analysis.
- *Data analysis* uses statistical measurements appropriate to data and goals. Frequency of analysis varies but must insure adequate numbers for data to be meaningful.
- *Analytical interpretation* involves using data to indicate threshold rates, clusters, outbreaks, or other events.
- *Utilizing results* must include specific steps that will be taken as a result of analytical interpretation. For example, if a threshold for infections is exceeded, clearly defined procedures should be outlined for dealing with that event.

Surveillance plans case-finding issues
Passive vs. active
A number of different issues must be resolved as part of the plans for surveillance, including active surveillance vs passive surveillance. . Passive surveillance, on the one hand, utilizes observations of medical and laboratory staff to identify and report infections, often requiring the staff to fill out a report and submit it. Passive surveillance often results in misclassification and delays as well as failure to report infections because no one is specifically charged with reporting. Staff involved in patient care

may not have or take the time to fill out reports. Active surveillance, on the other had, is a program specifically designed for finding nosocomial infections and using trained/certificated staff, such as infectious control personnel, whose primary purpose is infection control. Active surveillance tends to be more accurate and data more complete than passive surveillance because there is consistency and usually a more established program; however, active surveillance is also expensive because it requires dedicated staff.

Patient-based vs. laboratory-based
Surveillance plans may be patient-based or laboratory-based. *Patient-based* plans revolve around the patient, so the patient must be assessed for signs of infection, risk factors, quality of patient care, and staff compliance with infection control protocol. Patient-based plans are very time and staff intensive, requiring much time on the patient units in order to review charts, assess patient, and interview patient and staff. For large facilities, the cost of effective patient-based plans may be prohibitive. *Laboratory-based* plans, on the other hand, depend upon review of laboratory findings, often cultures, to determine if threshold rates have been exceeded. Laboratory findings are usually accurate, but the effectiveness of this type of plan depends on completeness of records and whether specimens are sent to the laboratory for analysis. If there are no clear protocols in place to determine when a specimen should be obtained, infections may be missed. This type of plan can utilize electronic monitoring systems, saving staff time.

Prospective vs. retrospective
Another issue that must be dealt with when deciding upon a plan for surveillance is whether the plan should be prospective or retrospective. *Prospective*, or concurrent, surveillance follows patients while they are hospitalized and includes the period after discharge to evaluate for surgical site infections. Because prospective surveillance is ongoing and continually evaluated, it can identify clusters of infection as they occur as well as ensuring that the infection control personnel have ongoing working relationships with other staff. When there appears to be an outbreak or cause for concern, analysis can be done fairly quickly. This is the type of surveillance required by those participating in the NNIS system. *Retrospective* surveillance, however, is done after the fact by a review of charts and records with no patient contact. There is often a time delay, then, between the time a problem presents and the time it is identified. This method is less expensive.

Surveillance methods
Incidence
Incidence and prevalence surveillance are both hospital-wide surveillance methods. *Incidence* surveillance is ongoing surveillance of infections of all hospitalized patients, recording the number of new infections in a population of patients over a specific period of time, so incidence surveillance is both time-consuming and expensive. However, it can identify clusters of infections and allows for risk-factor analysis. The incidence rate is calculated as follows:

$$\frac{(Numerator)}{(Demoniator)} = \frac{Number\ of\ new\ infections}{Total\ population\ in\ time\ period}$$

Prevalence
Prevalence surveillance involves both *period prevalence*, which is a specific pre-determined period of time for surveillance, and *point prevalence*, a specific point in time. Prevalence, then, is the number of case of nosocomial infections that are active during the period or point of time covered by the survey. The prevalence rate:

$$\frac{(Numerator)}{(Demoniator)} = \frac{Number\ with\ active\ infection}{Total\ population\ in\ time\ period}$$

Prevalence surveys are less time-consuming and expensive, but results can be skewed by random infections, resulting in overestimation.

Targeted surveillance
Targeted surveillance is limited in scope, focusing on particular types of infections, areas in the facility, or patient population. It is less expensive than hospital-wide surveillance and may provide more meaningful data, but clusters of infection outside the survey parameters may be missed. Targeted areas are picked based on characteristics such as frequency of infection, mortality rates, financial costs, and the ability to use date to prevent infections:

- *Site-directed* targets particular sites of infection, such as bloodstream, wound, or urine.
- *Unit-directed* targets selected service areas of the hospital, such as intensive care units or neonatal units.
- *Population-directed* targets groups that are considered high-risk, such as transplantation patients and those undergoing other invasive procedures.
- *Limited periodic* combines hospital-wide surveillance of all infections for one month each quarter followed by site-directed targets for the rest of the quarter. This increases the chance of detecting clusters of infection, but those that fall outside of the hospital-wide surveillance months would still be missed.

Priority-directed surveillance
Priority-directed surveillance is also referred to as surveillance by objective. It focuses on prioritizing efforts at infection surveillance in order to meet particular objectives. Serious infections are identified based on morbidity and mortality rates as well as costs and, importantly, the ability to effect preventive measures based on the data, so priority-directed surveillance is often directed at surgical site infections and pneumonia. Other infections are not simply ignored, but most resources are expended in focused areas.

Post-discharge surveillance
Post-discharge surveillance Post-discharge surveillance is conducted in a number of different manners; none standardized, and is more important with the decrease in the length of hospital stays, resulting in missing up to 50% of surgical site infections. Patients may be contacted directly through mailed questionnaires or by telephone. Sometimes physicians are contacted for information. Readmission data is evaluated, and in some cases, patients are followed in clinics or office visits. Data is often insufficient because of difficult with follow-up.

Targeted surveillance vs. hospital-wide
The major problem with hospital-wide surveillance is that cost is prohibitive, both in time and money; however, in order to detect all infections and to get a clear idea of the infection control problem of a facility, hospital-wide surveillance is necessary. When the CDC National Nosocomial Infections Surveillance system (NNIS) was initiated, it required hospital-wide surveillance but discontinued this in favor of targeted surveillance in 1999 because most hospitals couldn't afford more comprehensive surveillance. It is important that, even with the focus on targeted areas, infection control still does some hospital-wide surveillance because only about 20% of hospital-acquired infections occur in the ICU, the main targeted area. Additionally, only about 19% of hospital-acquired infections involve surgical sites. An electronic monitoring program that automatically monitors lab results can easily track all lab work. A rotating system of monitoring different units for specified periods of time can also be used to gain a more comprehensive picture of infections.

Identifying baseline rates

<u>Establishing threshold rates</u>
Threshold rates for infection control require a normal range so that variations below can indicate a decrease in infections or improvement in methods and above can trigger intervention. Establishing threshold rates must be done in each institution because it is extremely difficult to use data from facilities with different populations, different data collection methods, and different testing procedures. Thresholds may relate to particular types of tests or occurrences of infection per number of patients or patient days. The type of threshold to be established must be carefully defined. Establishing threshold rates involves a period of surveillance, which can be facility-wide but is often targeted to certain populations or procedures. This period may vary in length depending upon the size of the institution and other factors, but should be sufficient to provide adequate data. The data is compiled and evaluated and outbreak thresholds are then established. At this point, general surveillance is discontinued and surveillance is done related to those that exceed threshold.

<u>External benchmarking vs. internal trending</u>
External benchmarking involves analyzing data from outside an institution, such as monitoring national rates of hospital-acquired infection and comparing it to internal rates. In order for this data to be meaningful, the same definitions must be used as well as the same populations or effective risk stratification. Using NaSH data can be informative, but each institution is different, and relying on external benchmarking to select indicators for infection control can be misleading. Additionally, benchmarking is a compilation of data that may vary considerably if analyzed individually, further compounded by anonymity that makes comparisons difficult. Internal trending involves comparing internal infection rates of one area or population with another, such as ICU with general surgery, and this can help to pinpoint areas of concern within an institution, but making comparisons is still problematical because of inherent differences. Using a combination of external and internal data can help to identify and select indicators.

Notification system for Laboratory results

A notification system for the reporting of critical laboratory results should be made directly with the laboratory, if possible. Threshold rates should be derived first so that there is clarity about what results to report. If it's not possible to receive notification from the laboratory, then designated staff should be assigned to check lab results and report to the infection control personal. Notification should be done immediately so that intervention can begin. Infection control personnel should be available every day to receive notification. Notification may take various forms, depending upon the institution, staff, equipment, and resources:
- *Telephone:* Reports may be given directly to staff by phone.
- *Fax:* Reports may be faxed to the office of the infection control personnel.
- *Form:* A special form may be provided for notification purposes.
- *E-mail:* Use of electronic notification is especially useful if software is available that automatically triggers a notification when lab results exceed threshold rates.

Determining facility-specific denominator data

<u>Surgical procedures</u>
ASA scores
In 1961, the American Society of Anesthesiologists (ASA) established scores for assessment of the physical status of a patient prior to surgery. These scores are subjective and may be based on incomplete information, so they are not definitive. There are 6 categories:
1) *Normal* patient appears to be in good health.

- 56 -

2) *Systemic disease* is present but is mild.
3) *Systemic disease* is severe.
4) *Systemic disease* is life threatening.
5) *Moribund* patient will likely not survive without surgical intervention.
6) *rain-dead* patient whose surgery is for the purpose of harvesting organs.

The designation of "E" after the ASA score indicates that the surgical procedure is an emergency, defined as delay that might lead to loss of life or body part; however, this definition is narrow as surgery may be, for example, to correct severe pain. Category 5 is generally always classified as 5E because of the nature of the surgical need.

Wound classification
The traditional wound classification system classifies surgical wounds according to type and risk of infection:

- *Class I: Clean* wounds (risk <2%) do not enter an area of the body that is usually colonized by normal flora, such as the urinary or gastrointestinal tracts. There is primary closure and closed drainage, if necessary, with no break in aseptic technique.
- *Class II: Clean-contaminated* wounds (risk <10%) enter into colonized parts of the body, such as the respiratory or urinary tract, but surgery is elective and controlled rather than emergency. There is no indication of infection or break in aseptic technique.
- *Class III: Contaminated* wounds (risk 20%) have obvious inflammation but no purulent discharge. They may involve spillage of the gastrointestinal tract, penetrating wounds (<4 hours), and/or substantial break in aseptic technique.
- *Class IV: Dirty-infected* wounds (risk 40%) show obvious inflammation and purulent discharge. There may be perforation of viscera prior to surgery and/or penetrating wounds (>4 hours).

T-point classification system: The T-point classification system assigns time in hours based on information in the NNIS database about average length of surgery. The assigned T point for surgical procedures is the number of hours that equal the 75% percentile. Thus, a T point of 5 means that 75% of these types of surgery are completed within 5 hours. Exceeding the T point increases risk of infection or complications, so this system is used as one aspect of evaluation of surgical site infection risk although time is only one variable and should not be considered in isolation as other risk factors may be of more importance. The following are the T points for common surgical procedures:

Appendectomy	1
Hernia repair	2
Hysterectomy	2
Hip prosthesis	3
Vascular repair	3
Craniotomy	4
Coronary artery bypass graft	5

CDC/NNIS Risk Index System: The Centers for Disease Control and Prevention (CDC)/National Nosocomial Surveillance created the NNIS Risk Index System to standardize reporting of data regarding wound infections. This risk index integrates the traditional, T-point, and American Society of Anesthesiologists (ASO) classifications. The Risk Index scores range from 0-3 with a point for each of the applicable variables based on the other classifications:

0 point	No risk factors
1 point	Score of 3 or 4 on the traditional classification of wound that is contaminated or dirty

| 1 point | Score of 3, 4, or 5 on the ASO preoperative classification |
| 1 point | Exceeds the T point duration for this type of operation (>75%) |

Even with zero point, some risk of infection still exists, but the predictive percentage rate for surgical site infections increases with the Risk Index score:

Score	Will likely develop infection (percentage)
0 score	1.5%
1 score	2.9%
1 score	6.8%
1 score	13.0%

Surgical site infection definitions: Category I: Superficial incisional: Comparison of data requires that precise and standardized definitions be utilized for the descriptions of surgical cite infections. The CDC/NNIS developed the *CDC Definitions of Nosocomial Infections* to be used in reporting to NNIS and NaSH. The type of wound is classified according to these definitions, and then the Risk Index is applied to determine the severity of infection as well as rates of infection. Surgical site infections are identified by degree of infection among other criteria.

Category 1: The first category comprises *superficial incisional* infection, which occurs within 30 days of surgery and involves only skin and subcutaneous tissue of the incision. The patient has one of the following:
- o   Purulent drainage
- o   Organisms isolated from culture of wound fluid or tissue.
- o   Localized signs of infection, and wound is deliberately opened by physician, resulting in positive wound culture.
- o   Diagnosis of superficial infection by surgeon or attending physician.

Category 2: Deep incisional: The second category of the CDC/NNIS surgical site infection may include those wounds that have both superficial and deep incisional characteristics. The definition for the second category comprises *deep incisional* infections. These occur within 30 days of surgery if there is no implant or 1 year if an implant is in place. Infection appears related to the surgery and involves deep soft tissues (fascial and muscle layers) of the incision, and patient has one of following:
- o   Purulent drainage from incision but not organ/space component of surgical site.
- o   Spontaneous dehiscence of wound or deliberately opened by surgeon when patient has one of these symptoms: fever (38C), localized pain or tenderness, unless wound culture is negative.
- o   Abscess or other evidence of deep incision infection found on direct examination, histopathology or radiology.
- o   Diagnosis of a deep incisional infection by surgeon or attending physician.

Category 3: Organ/space: The third category of the CDC/NNIS surgical site infection definitions comprises *organ/space infections*, which occur within 30 days of surgery if no implant or 1 year if implant in place. Infection appears related to surgery and involves any part of the body, excluding the skin incision, fascia, or muscle layers, that is opened or manipulated during the operative procedure. Specific sites are assigned to organ/space SSI to further identify the location of the infection. Patient has one of the following:

- Purulent drainage from a drain that is placed through a stab wound into the organ/space.
- Organisms isolated from an aseptically obtained culture of fluid or tissue in the organ/space.
- An abscess or other evidence of infection involving the organ/space that is found on direct examination, during reoperation, or by histopathology or radiology.
- Diagnosis of an organ/space infection by a surgeon or attending physician

Surgeon-specific surgical procedures
Surgeon-specific data can be derived by limiting the denominator data to that surgeon's patient pool. The denominator number must be adequate (usually 100-1000) and the time of the survey of sufficient length to yield meaningful data, usually at least 4 weeks. Questions about both numerator and denominator data must be resolved. Will all surgical site infections be included together? Will superficial infections be surveyed separately from deep incisional or organ/space? Will adjustments for risk factors be made? Surgeon-specific data is rarely useful for comparison because of numerous variables. For example, two surgeons may do similar hip replacements, but one surgeon may specialize in sports injuries and deal with a younger, healthier population that the other surgeon whose patients are primarily elderly with chronic health problems. Infection rates may differ but, without adjusting for risk factors, the differences may be impossible to evaluate. Surgeon-specific data can be useful to help a surgeon implement changes to improve outcomes.

Rates of events calculations
When calculating rates of events (infection, death, disease), the formula requires a numerator, which is the targeted event (such as surgical site infections), and a denominator, which is the pool (such as the number of patients receiving surgery). The NaSH has established standardized numerator/denominator formulas. The procedure-associated formula:

Numerator	SSI infection
Denominator	Inpatients and outpatients undergoing operative
	Procedures
	Basic risk factor data for all procedures
	Specific risk factors for certain procedures

This new formula takes into account risk factors, which can include the ASO number, the wound classification, the T Point, or the Risk Index. The denominator data could include, for example, only those with ASO scores of 3, 4, or 5, but that ignores other variables. The results should be adjusted according to risk factor data. It is of critical importance that CDC definitions of infection be utilized for standardization.

Device related infections

Short-duration central lines
Short duration central lines are inserted <21-30 days for the purpose of administration of medicine, blood, fluids, and nutrition. Because they are invasive devices, they pose a risk of infection. Studies have shown that infection in short-duration devices is often caused by bacteria on the skin invading along the outside of the catheter. Different types of infections are common:
- Colonization of bacteria either on the outside or inside of the catheter may occur.
- Localized infection at the insertion site involves swelling, erythema, and discharge.
- Exit infection can occur where tunneled catheters exit the skin.

- o Tunnel infection occurs along the portion of the catheter that is tunneled under the skin before entering a vessel.
- o loodstream infections may be related to a catheter infection, with the same microbe, but they may occur as primary infections without evidence of local inflammation.

Long-term central lines

Long-term central lines are in place for >30 days and can cause a variety of infections, usually from microbes entering the catheter and moving down the inside to the bloodstream. There are 3 types of long-term central lines in common use. Non-tunneled catheters consist of subclavian silicone or peripherally-inserted central catheters (PICC). Tunneled catheters usually are inserted between the nipple and the sternum and have a Dacron cuff about 5 cm from the exit point. This cuff anchors the catheter to fibrous tissue. Implantable ports include a catheter and metal port, all inserted under the skin in a subcutaneus pocket, usually in the upper chest but sometimes in the arm. While infections may be similar to short-term central lines with the addition of port-pocket infection, of added concern is the development of biofilms that adhere to the catheters, leading to bloodstream infections and antibiotic resistance. The implantable port has a lower rate of infection than other types of lines.

Ventilators

Mechanical ventilation carries a risk of respiratory infection and pneumonia; usually from the patient's own microbes. Some infections are related to trauma and swelling that compromises tissue, resulting in aspiration of normal flora of the oropharyngeal area, and/or inhalation of microbes in aerosol form. Contaminated equipment may provide a reservoir for microbes, especially in moisture-containing tubes, nebulizers, or other equipment. Additionally, the ventilator essentially inoculates the respiratory tract with microbes. Nebulizers have been related to significant numbers of infection because the moist environment encourages colonization, especially if the nebulizers are reused for more than 48 hours. Humidifiers are often added to ventilators, but these tend to cause condensation in tubes, again providing fertile ground for microorganisms, unless heat moisture exchangers, which recycle exhaled heat and moisture, are used. Manual ventilator bags have been implicated in spread of infection because the inside of the bag wasn't sufficiently sterilized.

Urinary catheters

Urinary infections are the most common hospital-acquired infection in both acute and long-term care facilities, almost always caused by invasive devices, such as catheters and cystoscopes. Most people with continuous catheter drainage are chronically infected within 30 days. Catheters are frequently over-used and left in for too long, increasing risk of infection. Infections have occurred both in endemically and epidemically and may involve local inflammation, abscess formation, and, in males, infection can spread to the testes, prostate, and other reproductive organs. Because urinary tract infections are routinely treated with antibiotics, they have a role in increasing resistance of microorganisms to treatment. Fungal infections have increased markedly as a result. The urinary drainage bag serves as a reservoir for microorganisms, which can be transmitted on the hands of staff handling the bags. Contaminated bags can be implicated in pseudoinfections, where only the urine in the bag is infected.

Determining facility-specific denominator data for device related infections
The NaSH has established standardized numerator/denominator formulas. The device-associated formula:

Numerator	Selected device-associated infections
Denominator	Patient days
	Device days for selected event by location (ICU type)
	(Or by birth weight for high-risk neonates)

The population pool includes all those with infections related to specific devices, such as urinary catheters. Both the number of total patient days during the time period surveyed and the device days are recorded as a patient may be hospitalized for 6 days but have a catheter for only 4 days. Device days give more specific information. Data must be collected for sufficient time, at least 4 weeks, and in sufficient numbers to render useful data. Physician-specific data can be obtained, but should not be used for comparison. One physician may order urine cultures for all those with catheters and another physician may rarely do so. Since urinary infections are common with catheters, the physician who orders lab work may have higher statistics but actually a lower rate of infection.

Population-at-risk
Assessment of population is a very important component of a surveillance plan because each facility deals with a unique population. In this case, population refers to that segment of patients that will be studied because studying all patients, especially in large facilities, is impractical. Assessing population leads to targeted surveillance where particular areas, procedures, or types of patients are surveyed. Assessment includes:
- *Types of patients* should be evaluated, including whether or not they are medical or surgical and frequent diagnoses.
- *Procedures/treatments* should be assessed to determine those most commonly performed, especially those that are invasive.
- *Liability issues* must be considered in relation to those patients that affect liability and costs.
- *Community health issues*, such as outbreaks, may help to target populations.
- *Risk factors* for infection must be understood and used as part of assessment of needs.
- *Facility resources and support* must be considered because staff assistance is critical.

Resources
Resources must be utilized to properly assess populations for surveillance. Each facility will have different types of resources available, depending upon the size of the facility, the location, and the types of services it provides. A wide range of resources is often available:
- *Records* include individual medical records as well as summaries and reports from management and different medical units.
- *Risk management* at each facility is a good resource regarding the types of cases that involve liability and costs. Risk management may be able to target areas of concern.
- *Databases* for surgical procedures or other information may be available at institutions and should be analyzed.
- *Community health reports* from both public health and community agencies may have valuable information about community outbreaks and health concerns.
- *Human resources* should have health records and questionnaires regarding health problems and immunization records for staff.

Reviewing laboratory reports

In a small facility or targeted area of the hospital, reviewing all laboratory reports may be possible, but in larger facilities with multiple at risk populations, targeted review is more efficient. Computerized laboratory reporting systems that can flag particular pathogens or threshold rates facilitate the review of laboratory findings. "Alert" pathogens, those that are frequently implicated in hospital-acquired infections, such as *Staphylococcus aureus* and *Pseudomonas aeruginosa* should always be tagged for review. The infection control personnel reviewing laboratory reports should be familiar microbiology and with typical lab results for the complete blood count with the ability to recognize increases in leukocytes and differential shifts that may indicate infections. This person should also be knowledgeable about common hospital-acquired infections as well as those of particular concern for at risk populations in the facility related to outbreaks or breaches in infection control. Reports should be reviewed for unusual findings or clusters of infection.

Develop data collection forms

Surveillance and referral forms
Infection control programs depend upon the accuracy of data collection and the clarity of surveillance and referral forms. Forms should be developed after determining the approach that will be used, whether prospective or retrospective, and the focus of surveillance. Collection of information should be simplified and targeted just to surveillance objectives rather than broad-based generalized requests for referral information. Thus, forms may be developed for a number of different surveillance objectives. For example, the neonatal unit would have different surveillance objectives and different reporting forms than adult ICU. Staff involved in the use of the forms should be trained so that they understand the objectives and the type of information that is needed for data collection. Referral forms may be paper or electronic, depending upon the resources available in a facility. The duration of surveillance or points of surveillance should be clearly outlined. Forms may include questionnaires sent to particular staff or physician's office.

Computerized data forms

Pre-designed surveillance software packages
Managing data by hand can become quickly unwieldy. Standard spreadsheet software that is packaged with most PC can be used for simple reporting and data base functions but multiple variables are more difficult to manage. Using these programs often requires extensive programming and development. Utilizing pre-designed surveillance software packages can save time and expense and yield more accurate data. Statistical packages, such as SAS, SPSS, and MINITAB are available but require a steep learning curve. The CDC provides a free program, EpiInfo, which was originally designed for investigation of outbreaks but can be utilized to manage and analyze data. It consists of 5 separate programs: Nutstat (a nutritional program), MakeView to design data entry screens, Enter to enter data into screens designed with MakeView, Epimap to link data to maps, and Analysis for various types of statistical analysis. Commercial software programs specifically designed for infection control, such as AICE and EpiQuest, are also available.

Post discharge follow-up

If a communicable disease is identified as a possible source of infection, then the first step is to outline the epidemiology: the incubation period, the mode of transmission, the ease of transmission, and the symptoms. If the disease is reportable, then the local public health department must be notified immediately so that they can investigate and notify people. The physician should be notified as well as the patient or person with the communicable disease if they have not been informed. Next, a targeted retrospective survey must be done to identify those patients or staff who, because of time of hospitalization, bed proximity, contact, or shared use of equipment or facilities, may have contacted the disease. Physicians of patients should be notified and direct contact made with patients, preferably by telephone or in person if the disease poses a serious threat. If notification is sent by mail, follow up telephone calls should be done.

Integrating surveillance activities

Small acute hospitals
Because of accreditation requirements and health concerns, most small hospitals have infectious disease professionals (ICP), but they often have other duties as well. A minimum requirement for a team should include the ICP, a physician, an administrator, a pharmacist, and a laboratory representative. Unless laboratory reports are automated, routine review of laboratory findings must be done, but even in small facilities, review may be targeted to high-risk areas or populations. The ICP needs to train staff to assist in case finding and train all new hires in infection control procedures as well as giving regular in-service training to review procedures for other staff.   Surveillance must take into consideration the population of the facility and the purpose of surveillance so that data collection is meaningful and used for prevention. The ICP should maintain contact with the ICP from large feeder hospitals in the area and attend conferences and training with them when possible.

Long-term care facilities
The elderly often have decreased antibody-mediated and cell-mediated immune responses, leaving them less able to combat infections. Additionally, many elderly people suffer from malnutrition, which further impairs cell-mediated immunity. If patients have functional impairment, they may be dependent on staff for toileting and turning, and if not done adequately, patients can develop decubiti, increasing the chance of wound infection. Patients may have medical illnesses, such as circulatory impairment of diabetes that make them prone to infection. Invasive devices, such as feeding tubes and urinary catheters are used frequently, and infection is a common complication. Patients may be too weak to breathe deeply or cough so they are unable to clear bacteria from the respiratory tract. Another problem faced by the elderly is that their inflammatory response to infection is often altered, so they may exhibit fever without other symptoms, or they may exhibit no fever in the presence of infection, so diagnosis can be difficult.

Because people are being discharged early from acute care, many patients in long-term care facilities, especially nursing homes, may suffer from infection at the time of admission or may develop infection that began in the hospital but was undiagnosed. There are a number of infections that are quite common to long-term care facilities and should be targeted for surveillance.
- *Skin and soft tissue infections* can include surgical site infections, decubiti, bacterial or fungal infections, conjunctivitis, and scabies.
- *Respiratory infections* may range from common viral infections to pneumonia.
- *Urinary infections* are frequent because fluid intake is often inadequate and urinary catheters are often used for long-term control of incontinence.
- *Bloodstream infections* may be primary or secondary related to other infections, such as surgical site infection.
- *Gastrointestinal infections* may result in nausea, vomiting, and diarrhea. Bacterial infections can include *Shigella, Salmonella, E. coli,* and *Clostridium difficile.*

Long-term care facilities face many of the same challenges as small acute hospital in relation to infection control. Often infection control professionals have additional duties, but surveillance data is important

- 63 -

to identify problem areas and implement changes. The ICP from transferring acute hospitals should provide full information about transfer patients and serve as a resource. The facility ICP should check laboratory reports and interview patients and staff at least weekly to facilitate case finding. Incidence rates for targeted infections should be compiled. Education of staff is an important aspect of the ICPs duties because staff turnover in long-term care facilities is high. Staff often begins work with little training or knowledge of infection control, especially nurses aids who may provide the primary patient care. All staff needs to be trained in infection control so that they can assist in case finding and institute preventive measures. Because urinary infections are common, many patients receive antibiotics, so antibiotic review should be ongoing.

Home health

Home health patients have many of the same types of infections found in both acute and long-term care facilities. Invasive devices, such as central lines, nasogastric, and tracheotomy tubes all predispose patients to opportunistic infections that may be localized or systemic. Vascular access devices are a common cause of infection especially if hygiene is not rigorous with the patient and caregivers. Urinary infections are common, especially if urinary catheters are used. Caregivers in the home often must handle and empty drainage bags and can easily spread contamination.   Respiratory infections are common for a variety of reasons: patients may not follow through on deep breathing, coughing, and exercise programs. Ventilation and dialysis equipment may not be cleaned or changed as frequently as it should be. Patients often reuse equipment that is clearly indicated for single use only because of costs or inconvenience involved in getting new equipment, again leading to infection.

There is much that cannot be controlled in the home environment, so staff face challenges in surveillance even while the numbers of home care patients and the severity of illness of these patients is increasing. Many patients have invasive medical devices, sometimes multiple. About 20% of patients already have infections when admitted to home health care. The ICP, often a staff person with other duties, is dependent on others for much data: the acute hospital, the laboratory, the physician, and the patient. Surveillance in the home often involves weekly reports completed by staff other than the ICP. Much of the ICP's focus must be on facilitating case finding by training staff and preparing reporting forms. Additionally the ICP must assure that protocols for home care are followed, including cleansing of equipment and changing of invasive devices according to a schedule. Any indications of infection must be reported to the patient's physician.

Risk stratification

Risk stratification involves statistical adjustment to account for confounding and differences in risk factors. Confounding issues are those that confuse the data outcomes, such as trying to compare different populations, different ages, or different genders. For example, if there are two physicians and one has primarily high-risk patients, and the other has primarily low risk patients, the same rate of infection (by raw data) would suggest that the infection risks are equal for both physicians' patients. However, high risk patients are much more prone to infection, so in this case risk stratification to account for this difference would show that the patients of the physician with low risk patients had a much higher risk of infection, relatively-speaking. Risk stratification is also used to predict outcomes of surgery by accounting for various risk factors (including ASO score, age, and medical conditions). Risk stratification is an important element of data analysis.

Communicable diseases requiring follow-up and isolation

Types of surveillance
There are four types of surveillance that can be utilized:

- *Admitting history/admission physical* can help to identify high-risk behaviors or symptoms that may not be current but can indicate a communicable disease. Questioning answers to elicit more information is also helpful.
- *dmitting diagnosis* serves as a key element to determine if further evaluation should be done, especially if the diagnosis is a common opportunistic infection involving particular infectious diseases. For example, cytomegalovirus is often related to HIV infection.
- *Symptoms*, such as chronic or severe cough or diarrhea, should trigger further investigation to determine if there is a contagious cause.
- *Laboratory review* should be ongoing after threshold rates are established for different lab tests. Any abnormality that is suggestive of an infectious disease process should be evaluated to determine if further follow-up or isolation is needed.

Antimicrobial monitoring and evaluation

ntimicrobial monitoring and evaluation is an important aspect of infection control and reduction of antibiotic resistance. A program must be implemented that includes a protocol for use and education for staff. Typical monitoring includes:

- *Antibiotic protocols* for use should include a formulary and guidelines for specific hospital units or patient populations. These protocols must be monitored regularly and updated as needed, with rotation of antibiotics is indicated. Use and effectiveness of antibiotics must be monitored on an ongoing basis. Guidelines should include steps to take if the first line antibiotics are not effective.
- *Laboratory testing* should help to determine the most effective antibiotic control for significant isolates so that treatment is targeted and effective.
- *Stop orders* should be in place in the pharmacy to ensure that antibiotics are ordered for the correct duration of time.
- *Prophylaxis protocols* with specific doses and durations should be established for short-term use of antibiotics in particular circumstances, such as preoperatively.

1996 CDC isolation guidelines

Through the years, the CDC has issued a number of different guidelines for isolation precautions. The 1996 CDC isolation guidelines were an update from the "Universal precautions" guidelines that dealt with blood and some body fluids but did not directly address other types of transmission. There are now 2 tiers of isolation precautions.

Tier I, standard precautions

Tier I deals with standard precautions that should be in place for all patients. *Standard precautions* include protection from all blood and body fluids and include the use of gloves, face barriers, and gowns as needed to avoid being splashed with fluids. Hand washing remains central to infection control and should be with plain (not antimicrobial) soap or instant antiseptic. Private rooms are used for those who contaminate the environment (uncontrolled diarrhea, cough, etc.) or are unhygienic. If no private room is available, patients with the same type of infection, same colonizing organism, may share a room.

Tier II, transmission-based precautions, airborne and droplet

Tier II of the CDC isolation guidelines protects from three types of transmission. The first type provides protection from diseases spread by small airborne droplets (<5mm), including measles, tuberculosis, and varicella. *Airborne precautions* include placing patient in a private room with monitored negative airflow and the door closed. People who are susceptible to the disease, such as those not immune against measles, should not enter the room. Respiratory precautions (a mask) should be worn if the patient has suspected or confirmed tuberculosis. Patient should wear mask outside of room.

The second type provides protection from diseases spread by large airborne droplets (>5mm), easily spread by talking, coughing, or sneezing, but do not travel more than 3 feet. Diseases include viral influenza, pertussis, streptococcal pharyngitis or pneumonia, *Neisseria* meningitides, and mumps.

Droplet precautions include private room. Staff and visitors who are within 3 feet of the patient must wear masks, and the patient must wear a mask outside of room.
The 1996 CDC isolation guidelines: Tier II, transmission-based precautions, contact.

Tier II of the CDC Isolation guidelines includes the third type, contact, which provides protection from diseases spread by direct hand-to-hand or skin-to-skin contact, such as those with significant infection or colonization and those who have suspected or confirmed multi-drug resistance, which may include vancomycin-resistant *Enterococci* and *Staphylococcus aureus.*

Contact precautions include placing the patient in a private room or room with someone with the same infection. Gloves should be used as for standard precautions but should immediately be removed and hands sanitized after contact with infective material. A clean protective gown should be worn inside the room for close contact with patient, including caring for a patient who is incontinent or has uncontained drainage. The patient should not leave the room if possible and equipment should be dedicated for patient use or disinfected before use by other patients.

Some diseases may require some combination of airborne, droplet, and contact precautions: Lassa fever, Marburg virus, and smallpox.

Evaluating surveillance plans
Surveillance should be done with a goal in mind, and the data collected should be used as a basis to plan strategies of intervention or to identify indicators for further study. One measure, then, of the effectiveness of a surveillance plan is the degree to which it has initiated changes or increased efficiency. The effectiveness of the plan should be evaluated on a regular basis, reviewing not only the type of surveillance but also the targets, as this may need to be changed, especially if there is evidence of outbreaks or changing patterns of infections that are unaccounted for. Laboratory findings are an integral part of surveillance and these findings should be reviewed as part of the overall evaluation as often the first indication of an outbreak is reflected in laboratory results. Threshold rates may require adjustment or additions in order to facilitate case finding. Questionnaires and interviews can help to evaluate effectiveness of surveillance.

Collection of Surveillance Data

A systematic approach to record surveillance data requires planning and consistency. Surveillance may involve questionnaires, medical records, or electronic review.

- *Questionnaires* should be standardized and designed to obtain information that is quantifiable when possible. Questions should be clear, unambiguous, and non-threatening. Open-ended questions may be appropriate for some types of information gathering, especially in relation to information that may be embarrassing.
- *Coding* of data collection should be consistent, with specific codes for units, populations, and/or individuals to facilitate analysis. Thus, the report of a patient with a cough would have the same identification code as the laboratory work for that patient.
- *Medical record review* should be systematic and targeted as much as possible. Reporting forms should be utilized that include all necessary information in one form.

- *Electronic surveillance* should involve use of threshold data reports that are generated should be directly integrated with the data analysis system.

Standardized definitions

Abbreviations
The following abbreviations are commonly used in infection control:
dV: Adenovirus
SA: American Society of Anesthesiologists
KV: BK virus
SI: Blood stream infection.
CDC: Centers for Disease Control & Prevention
CMV: Cytomegalovirus
CVC: Central venous catheter
CVL: Central venous line
EPA: Environmental protection agency
FDA: Food and Drug Administration
HAV: Hepatis A virus
HBV: Hepatitis B virus
HCV: Hepatitis C virus
HEPA: High efficiency particulate air [filter]
HHV-6: Human Herpesvirus-6
HSV: Herpes simplex virus
HIV: Human immunodeficiency virus
ICP: Infection control professional
JCV: JC virus
MRSA: Methicillin-resistant Staphylococus aureus.
NaSH: National Surveillance System for Healthcare Workers
NHSN: National Healthcare Safety Network
NIOSH: National Institute for Occupational Safety and Health (CDC)
NNIS: National Nosocomial Infections Surveillance System
OSHA: Occupational Safety and Health Administration (U.S. Department of Labor)
PICC: Peripherally-inserted central catheters
SSI: Surgical site infection
TPN: Total parenteral nutrition
UTI: Urinary tract infection
VRE: Vancomycin-resistant *Enterococcus*
VCV: Varicella-Zoster virus

CDC definitions
In 1988, the CDC established the "CDC Definitions for Nosocomial Infections" to standardize reporting and obtain meaningful data for a national database. The definitions include:
- *Infection site:* For example, a urinary tract infection is coded as UTI and a surgical site infection is coded as SSI.
- *Code:* The site of infection is further coded according to the sub-type: SUTI, systematic urinary tract infection: ASB, asymptomatic bacteriuria; and OUTI, other infections of the urinary tract.
- *Definition:* The definition of the infection outlines the criteria for inclusion into a coded category. For example, UTI-SUTI (urinary tract infection—systematic urinary tract infection) includes 4 different criteria. For example, Criterion 1 is defined as:

o   Patient has at least 1 of the following signs or symptoms with no other recognized cause: fever (>38°C), urgency, frequency, dysuria, or suprapubic tenderness AND patient has a positive urine culture, that is $\geq 10^5$ microorganisms per cm^3 of urine with no more than 2 species of microorganisms.

Identification and classification of events, indicators, or outcomes

In order for comparison data, internal or external, to be valid, there must be consistency in definitions as to what comprises a nosocomial infection, including onset, symptoms, and laboratory findings. Clear definitions must be in place for events, indicators, and outcomes.

- *Events* are most commonly defined according to the CDC definitions for nosocomial infections, but in some cases other definitions may be developed, but they must be used consistently and cannot then be compared to events using other definitions.
- *Indicators* are used as a measure of quality because they represent numerator data, that is the number of events that are being targeted, such as specific types of infections, defined as narrowly as possible. The denominator data, in this case, is the population at risk for the indicator event.
- *Outcomes* are measurements of indicators, such as the number of infections per a specified denominator, such as100 patient days, or 1000 device day. Outcomes should provide feedback.

Collecting and compiling data

Surgical procedures

The collection of data for surgical procedures may vary according to the size and resources of the institution. Data may be collected and compiled from operative schedules, operative reports, laboratory results, medical records, and reports of antibiotic use. Data may be collected for targeted populations. If data are collected for all surgeries performed, then the results need to be stratified to account for different risk factors, such as the type of surgery, the ASO score, the wound classification, and the T point. Surgeon-specific data should be provided as feedback to the individual surgeons rather than used as a basis of comparison. Some studies have indicated that providing feedback has successfully reduced rates of infection, but other studies have been inconclusive because of differences in variables. If possible, data collection should be electronically automated. Using an automated database that includes such information as the ASO score, T point, Risk Index, and codes for procedures can facilitate accurate collection of data.

Surgical site infections

With the increase in antibiotic resistance, the use and timing of antibiotics are becoming of critical importance, and collection of data correlating pre-, intra-, and peri-operative antibiotic use to correlate with surgical site infections can provide valuable outcome information to be used for planning and intervention. In this case, the numerator data is defined as the type of antibiotic use. One problem encountered is gaining adequate data because some pre-surgical and peri-surgical antibiotics will be prescribed outside of the hospital so data may be dependent on questionnaires or interviews. Denominator data will be the population of those with surgical site infections. Again, some infections may not be evident until after discharge, so follow up with patients and doctors is necessary if the correlations are to have validity. Additionally, the denominator data may be stratified according to various risk factors, such as type of surgery, ASO score, generating different data according to risk factors.

Device utilization

Two common risk factors for hospital-acquired infections are length of stay and days of device utilization, including central lines, urinary catheters, and ventilators. The longer the invasive device is in place, the more likely an infection will occur, so collecting data on use and duration of invasive devices is especially important for infection control. Device records should be kept for each population or unit (such as ICU, HRN), electronically if possible. Coded information should be readily available and include the type of illness or procedure, the type of invasive device, the dates and duration of use, and indications of infection. It's important that data be kept for use of all invasive devices, not just occurrences of device-related infection, because the total number of invasive device days becomes the denominator data and it's impossible to arrive at meaningful indicator data and outcomes without this information.

Populations at risk
Populations at risk must be defined for each institution, usually on the basis of an initial surveillance. There is no single way to define a population at risk; some procedures pose more risks than other: transplant surgery versus appendectomies. Some units in the hospital are associated with higher risk: ICUs versus general medical floors. Targeting specific high-risk populations simplifies the collection of data by limiting surveillance and concentrating resources. Data collection should be stratified initially, if possible, so that information about populations and sub-populations is separated because this facilitates analysis and helps to identify outbreaks or deviations. For example, ICU data should not be commingled with high-risk nursery HRN data because the populations have completely different risk factors and expected outcomes. Electronic collection of data simplifies this process, but collecting data from questionnaires, interviews, lab reports, and medical records, while more time-consuming, can suffice.

Data from other agencies

Data from other departments or agencies can be very useful for the collection of surveillance data. The admissions department collects demographic information as part of the basic admissions questionnaire. For example, information about where a patient resides or was born can yield important risk factors, especially if diseases, such as malaria or Chagas disease, are endemic to these areas. This information is especially important if there is a large immigrant population. Additionally, data from public health departments about community-acquired infections or risks can trigger changes in surveillance in the hospital to reflect public health concerns. Some diagnoses of infections are based on clinical findings rather than laboratory results, and the pharmacy can be a valuable resource, providing information about the use of medications, primarily antibiotics, which may indicate treatment for infection. Operative reports can be used to identify high-risk populations, as not all patients will be treated in high-risk areas, such as ICUs.

Computerized systems

The use of a computerized system for entering data can pose a number of problems because often systems in use are not integrated, so the lab reports and medical records may be on incompatible systems. There are a number of different ways to enter data:
- *Manual data entry* is probably the most common method. This can involve charting directly into the computer or copying information, such as lab reports, after the fact. The responsibility for entering data must be clearly outlined to prevent a backlog. Staff must be thoroughly trained in the correct procedures for data entry.
- *Scanners* can be programmed to read particular forms, such as those with boxes marked. Text can also be scanned so that reports from outside the system can be added.
- *PDAs* can be used to copy data for transfer rather than entering data on forms by hand.

Compiling Surveillance Data

Determining the incidence of nosocomial infections

Adult and pediatric ICU component and high-risk nursery
Compilation of data to determine incidence of nosocomial infection may be sentinel-based, which is related to a breakdown in infection control and utilizes raw data regarding events, or population-based (the most common), which requires both numerator and denominator data. Population-based data compilation is usually done following guidelines and definitions provided by the CDC, NaSH. One or more of the CDC surveillance components may be used, but once chosen, data must be collected for a minimum of one month. In each case, the numerator data is the number of nosocomial infections:

- *Adult and Pediatric ICU component* may use as denominator data the number of patients at risk, total patient days, or total days of invasive device use. Data may be compiled for specific sites.
- *High Risk Nursery component* uses denominator data as for adult and pediatric ICU but statistics are compiled according to birth weight:
  - <1000 g
  - -1500 g
  - -2500 g
  - ≥ 2500 g

Surgical patient component and antimicrobial use and resistance (AUR)
The CDC surveillance components are not necessarily mutually exclusive. For example, surgical patients may also be in ICU:

- *Surgical patients component* includes 8 different operative procedures that can be followed according to the plan of the facility. All patients undergoing the selected operative procedure(s) are surveyed to for either surgical site infections or all infections. Risk factors are accounted for in the statistical analysis.
- *Antimicrobial use and resistance (AUR) component* compiles data from 3 or more areas: 1) ICU or specialty area, such as a transplant unit, 2) all combined patient areas, excluding ICUs, and 3) all combined outpatient areas. Data about the use of antimicrobials and resistance is compiled. This component is the only one that does not require compilation of infection rates, but the CDC recommends that the ICU chosen for AUR surveillance be the same used for surveillance of ICU infections so some infection data is generated.

Incidence
The incidence of nosocomial infections is the number of new occurrences of infections (numerator data) in a population at risk (denominator data) during a specific time period that is the same for both numerator and denominator. The *incidence rate* is the number of events (numerator) divided by the number of the population at risk (denominator), often expressed as the number of infections per 100 patients. Incidence may also be used to calculate *incidence density*, which is the rate at which disease occurs in relation to the size of the population without disease. Incidence density uses the number of infections (numerator) in relation to units of time (denominator), such as the number of infections that occur in 1000 patient days. Incidence may also be used to calculate attack rate, expressed as a percentage of an at-risk population that is infected. The attack rate is used to calculate incidence rates during outbreaks of specific populations.

Calculating device-related infections

Device-related infections are usually calculated by using the number of infection events (numerator) in relation to either the number of insertions/uses or the number of device days (denominator). For example, calculation the number of urinary infections per catheter insertions would be expressed as 1.4 per 100 insertions. Infections calculated using device days are done by adding together the total device days of the target population:

Patient A	4 days with the device
Patient B	6 days
Patient C	10 days
Patient D	7 days
Total device days	27 days

Assuming there was one infection (numerator) during these 27 device days (denominator), the rate would be 0.37 multiplied by 1000 (the scale factor), resulting in an estimate of 37 infections per 1000 device days. Of course, a sample should involve far more than 4 patients and 27 days for the calculations to be statistically meaningful.

Basic statistical techniques

Measures of averages
Measures of averages locate the center point of a group of data:
- *Mean* is the average number. However, since distribution can vary widely, the mean may not give an accurate picture. For example, if compiling data and one unit has 20 infections per 100 and the other has 1 infection per 100, the mean (21÷2) is 10.5 per 100, which has little validity.
- *Median* is the 50th percentile. For example, consider the following numbers: 1, 3, 7, 9, and 15. The number 7 is the median (middle) number. If there were an even number, the 2 middle numbers would be averaged: 1, 3, 7, 9, 14, and 15. The numbers 7 and 9 are averaged so the median is 8. If there is an even distribution, the mean and median will be the same. The wider the difference between the two, the more uneven the distribution.
- *Mode* is the number occurring with the highest frequency. There may be bi-modal or tri-modal numbers.

Measures of distribution
Measures of distribution show the spread or dispersion of data.
- *Range* is the distance from the highest to the lowest number. The term interquartile is used in infection control to denote the range between the 25th percentile and the 75th percentile. Range is usually reported with median to provide information about both the center point and the dispersion.
- *Variance* measures the distribution spread around an average value. It is often used to calculate the effect of variables. A large variance suggests a wide distribution and a small variance indicates that the random variables are close to the mean.
- *Standard deviation* is the square root of the variance and shows the dispersion of data above and below the mean in equally measured distances. In a normal distribution, 68% of the data is within one deviation (measured distance) of the mean, 95% within 2 deviations and 99.7% within 3 deviations.

Calculating Rates and Ratios

A rate is the number of events per a given population (a rate of 3 infections per 100 patients) or per a time period (a rate of 3 infections per 1000 device days). These figures are expressed as the ratios

3:100 and 3:1000. Rates and ratios are accessible, and much infection control data is expressed by these statistics. However, data should be stratified, taking risk factors into account, and different rates derived for different populations for validity. Risk ratio is the ratio of incidence of infection among those who have been exposed compared to the incidence among those who have not been exposed. A risk ratio of 1.0 suggests that there is equal risk of infection. A higher number suggests the probability that those exposed will have higher rates. Thus, a number of 1.5 shows that the exposed group is 1.5 times more likely to become infected than those not exposed. A lower number suggests exposure brings less risk of infection (immunity).

Prevalence of epidemiologically significant findings

While incidence counts new infections diagnosed during a time period, prevalence (proportion) counts existing infections, regardless when the disease was contracted, during a specified period of time (period prevalence) or at a point in time (point prevalence). Prevalence is a good measure of the overall burden of infections on a facility, expressing how common infections are. Prevalence is often expressed as a percentage. In *limited-duration prevalence,* prevalence is looked at retrospectively. That is, it counts all those alive at a point in time who, during a prescribed duration of time (past 5 years, for example), had a particular disease. *Complete/lifetime prevalence*, on the other hand, counts all those alive at a particular point in time who had the disease at any time in the past or present, whether cured or in current treatment, usually expressed as a ratio of those with the disease compared to a given population.

Antiobiotic resistance patterns

Data to monitor antibiotic resistance patterns may be compiled with one or two different types of data. Antibiotic resistance patterns may be surveyed for a given population through various cultures (sputum, blood, or urine) to which antibiotic sensitivities are completed. Organisms that are typically monitored include:
- Vancomycin resistant *Enterococci*
- Drug resistant *Streptococcus pneumoniae*
- Methicillin-resistant *Staphylococcus aureus*
- Drug resistant Group A *Streptococci*

Resistance patterns may also be correlated with antibiotic use. First antibiotic use must be monitored in relation to infections, whether the antibiotics were prescribed prophylactically before or during surgery/ exposure or in response to an infection. Then cultures must be taken of the target population and antibiotic sensitivity testing completed. Monitoring antibiotic resistance patterns is often part of establishing a formulary or protocols for antibiotic use. The increasing prevalence of antibiotic resistance poses a major concern for healthcare providers and is a primary concern of infection control.

Controlling and decreasing antibiotic resistance
There are a number of strategies that are employed to attempt to control and decrease antibiotic resistance because poor practice in the administration of antibiotics coupled with inadequate infection control have resulted in increasingly antibiotic-resistant microorganisms. Strategies include:
- ntibiotic formulary restricting use: Studies have demonstrated that only about 50% of antibiotic use is appropriate. A formulary lists appropriate antibiotics, including dosage and duration, for different conditions and situations. Usually a procedure must be followed to justify alternate therapy.

- Cycling of antibiotics: Cycling involves a rotating list of antibiotics, within or between classes, to be used. Studies have indicated that, for multiple reasons, the "off" cycle drugs are frequently still used and optimal durations (usually 1-4 months) between cycling are still being studied.
- Combination antibiotic therapy: Studies have demonstrated that pairing two antibiotics, such as an older with a newer variety, can treat resistant strains.

Genetic components

ntibiotic resistance is a major area of concern in infection control because of a marked increase in recent years, leading to concern that increasing numbers of microorganisms, especially bacteria, may become resistant to all antibiotics. Antibiotic use can result in **genetic changes** that result in antibiotic resistance. These changes include:

- *Foreign DNA* can be introduced with gene transfers from one type of bacteria to another via plasmids (circular, double strands of DNA that can replicate in a cell but are separate from chromosomal DNA), which carry genes for resistance. Others are able to acquire DNA from the environment.
- *Mutations*, even very minor ones, can select for resistance to antibiotics by altering sensitivity or binding sites.
- *Cross-resistance* occurs when changes in sensitivity to one antibiotic provides resistance to other antibiotics as well.
- *Co- resistance* occurs when multiple mechanisms of resistance are present in the same microorganism.

Primary mechanisms

There are a number of **mechanisms** by which bacteria are resistant to antibiotics. The antibiotic-bacteria combination, dosage, and duration of therapy all affect the type of resistance. These resistant bacteria have genes in their DNA or plasmids that control protective mechanisms:

- *Inactivation* occurs when the bacteria secrete different enzymes that chemically modify the antibiotics, such as penicillin and chloramphenicol. This is the primary method of antibiotic resistance.
- *Iteration of blinding sites* may involve changes removal of molecules in the cell wall, preventing the antibiotics, such as vancomycin and methicillin, from attaching to the bacteria.
- *Efflux pumps* essentially are mechanisms in the bacteria that serve as pumps to force antibiotics, such as tetracycline and quinolones, out of the cell.
- *Alteration of cell wall* through alterations of proteins eliminates ports of entry into the bacteria cell wall by decreasing permeability.

Interpretation of Surveillance Data

Generation, analysis and validation of surveillance data

Most generation of data is from available resources, such as admissions records, questionnaires, interviews, medical records, public health reports, and laboratory reports. In some cases, creating data is part of the surveillance process. For example, urine cultures may be done routinely as part of a surveillance plan, or threshold rates may generate further testing. Analysis should be done in a timely manner, especially important for the detection of outbreaks. The type of analysis will depend upon the expected outcomes and the purpose of surveillance. Validation of data is an ongoing process. All steps in the generation and analysis of data should be reviewed regularly, especially when threshold rates have been exceeded. If, for example, there is an apparent outbreak of antibiotic resistant bacteria detected sputum cultures, then the procedures for obtaining the specimens as well as laboratory procedures need to be validated to ensure that the outbreak is not a pseudo-epidemic caused by faulty lab procedures or other deviations in infection control.

Preparing periodic reports of analyzed data

Reports should be generated by the infection disease professional on a regular basis, which may vary from monthly to quarterly or even annually, depending upon the size of the institution and the population numbers or device days. Statistics must include adequate denominator data for meaningful analysis, and this can require a longer period of time. Specific data about individual patients or healthcare workers are often protected by laws regarding privacy, so information about individuals cannot be disseminated unless anonymity can be assured. Reports to individual physicians about their own infections rates should be provided confidentially and comparison rates done without identifying physicians. Reports are usually presented to the infection control committee, but reports should also be presented to staff in areas of survey. Thus, if a study involved an ICU, the ICU staff and physicians should be aware of the study results so that they can evaluate the effectiveness of infection control procedures or institute preventive methods.

Comparison of rates
Reports of hospital-acquired infections are often used as a basis of comparison between one facility and others or one department in a facility, such as an ICU, and another, such as a transplant unit. Even in-house comparisons must be interpreted carefully because a higher rate of infection does not always mean patients are at increased risk. Numerous factors must be accounted for if a comparison is to be meaningful:
- *Definitions* must be uniform and consistent, following CDC definitions or specific definitions that have been developed for the population at risk or facility.
- *Protocols* for data collection should be uniform so that data is collected in the same way in different units, and case finding should be consistent and accurate. There should also be consistency in obtaining supporting laboratory tests.
- *Risk factors* should be similar or results stratified to account for differences in risk factors.

Computerized systems to analyze data

The analysis of data by hand is impractical and time-consuming unless the surveyed population is very small. Most statistical analysis is done using computer software programs that automatically analyze the data in a number of different ways and can account for risk factors. Software programs have various other utilizations. They may be used to generate not only numeric data and text reports but also various graphs. The amount and type of data that must be entered into a program varies according to the type of software and the necessary data for reports that will be generated. If different programs are used to collect and analyze data, then the ability to move data from one program to another may be necessary in order to generate reports. Data-entry design is important: data to which mathematical calculations are done is entered as numeric data, but some numbers (telephone and Social Security) to which no mathematical calculations are done, are entered as text data.

Identifying variances from baseline data

Identification of variances from baseline data first requires baseline data that is representative for the target population. This involves an initial period of surveillance and review. Baseline data can be established for various periods of time, but a 1-month period is commonly used. Threshold rates should also be established. Once the baseline is established, new data is analyzed to determine if there are variances (changes), usually increases although decreases may be identified if data is collected for the purpose of charting improvements. The basis for an alert should be predetermined. For example, if infection rates increase 2 standard deviations above the monthly mean, this may trigger an alert. Alerts may be tied to time so that increases over a 3-month period trigger alerts. Once data triggers a variance alert, then statistical analysis must be completed to determine the relevancy of the variance, the probability of it having occurred by chance, in order to determine if the variance has statistical significance.

Statistical significance

p values
One problem with surveillance data is that sometimes there can be variations in data by chance alone, so a sudden increase in incidence of infection may not indicate an outbreak but rather a normal statistically acceptable variation. The p value calculates the probability that the results occurred by chance. *P* values are expressed in a range from >0 to 1.0.
- <0.05 is statistically significant with only a <5% probability that the event could have occurred by chance, and conversely a 95% chance the event is significant.
- >5% is considered not statistically significant, probably occurring by chance.

It's important to realize that p value alone is not enough to make a determination that an event is of no significance because, for example, a limited outbreak may not generate enough data to show significance, but it can still be epidemiologically important. The p value is just one measurement of evidence and should be combined with other statistical analyses.

Causal inference/Hill's criteria
In epidemiology, a statistical association is not necessarily definitive. Sir A. Bradford Hill (1897-1991), who made important contributions to research methods related to epidemiology, developed criteria to judge a causal inference. The more criteria are met, the more likely that an association is causal; that is, an exposure caused a disease.
- *Strength of association* as measured by the p value <0.05.
- *Temporality:* Cause must precede event.
- *Consistency of observations:* The same effect occurs in different populations and settings.
- *Plausibility of theory:* The theory is based on sound biologic principles.
- *Coherence:* The theory does not conflict with other knowledge/theories.
- *Specificity:* One primary cause for an outcome strengthens causality.
- *Dose relationship:* An increase in exposure should increase the risk.
- *Experimental evidence:* Related experimental research may increase the causal inference.
- *Analogical extension:* That which is true in one situation may apply to another.

Bias
Selection bias occurs when the method of selecting subjects results in a cohort that is not representative of the target population because of inherent error in design. For example, if all patients who develop urinary infections with urinary catheters are evaluated per urine culture and sensitivities for microbial resistance, but only those patients with clinically-evident infections are included, a number of patients with sub-clinical infections may be missed, skewing the results. Selection bias is only a concern when participants in studies are specifically chosen. Many surveillance studies do not involve selection of subjects.

Information bias occurs when there are errors in classification, so an estimate of association is incorrect. Non-differential misclassification occurs when there is similar misclassification of disease or exposure among both those who are diseased/exposed and those who are not. Differential misclassification occurs when there is a differing misclassification of disease or exposure among both those who are diseased/exposed and those who are not.

Hospital reporting

There are a number of issues related to hospital reporting that can result in inaccurate data.

- *Insufficient information* may be the result of incomplete medical records or lab reports at the time of survey. There may be a failure in the reporting procedure so that some data is not reported.
- *Evaluation errors* may occur even when data is available but is overlooked or the significance is not understood so that the data is not included in a survey.
- *Insufficient laboratory testing* is a frequent finding of studies. Very often indications of infection are clinically evident but cultures that would verify infection are not ordered by the physician or are not automatically triggered by established threshold rates.
- *Negligence* may relate to reluctance to verify and report infections in order to keep infection rates low.

Because of differences in efficiency of collecting data, the facility with the lowest infection rate may be the one with the least accurate collection of data.

Internal and external validity

Many surveillance plans are most concerned with internal validity, adequate unbiased data properly collected and analyzed within the population studied, but studies that determine the efficacy of procedures or treatments, for example, should have external validity as well; that is, the results should be generalizable (true) for similar populations. Replication of the study with different subjects, researchers, and under different circumstances should produce similar results. For various reasons, some people may be excluded from a study so that instead of randomized subjects, the subjects may be highly selected so when data is compared with another population in which there is less or more selection, results may be different. The selection of subjects, in this case, would interfere with external validity. Part of the design of a study should include considerations of whether or not it should have external validity or whether there is value for the institution based solely on internal validation.

Time-related risk and multiple events

Most studies of hospital-acquired infections involve time at risk rather than patient numbers, so studies of *incidence density* related to invasive devices, such as intravenous lines or urinary catheters, are often based the number of infections per 1000 device days, that is days at risk. If there are 200 patients with a total of 600 device days and 6 patients develop infections, those 6 patients are no longer "at risk" because they have the infection and become part of the numerator data (number of infections), so their device days counted only up to the point where an infection is diagnosed. Additionally, frequently the same patient may have multiple or recurring infections, with the first infection a significant risk factor for the second. Generally, first events only are included in the data to avoid counting a subject more than once. Alternately, data may be stratified according to the number of infections to calculate risks. Longitudinal studies that account for multiple infections over time may also be completed.

Using tables, graphs and charts to present reports

Presenting data in the form of charts and graphs provides a visual representation of the data that is easy to comprehend. There are basically 3 types of graphs: line, bar, and pie.

- *Line graphs* have an x and y axis, so they are used to show how an independent variable affects a dependent variable. Line graphs can show a time series with time usually on the x (horizontal) axis. This graph might be used to show number of infections per week/month.

- *Bar graphs* are used to compare and show the relationship between two or more groups. The graphs can show quantifiable data as bars that extend horizontally, vertically, or stacked. Bar graphs might be used to show comparison data of different populations or to compare data from one time period to another.
- *Pie charts* are used to show what percentage an item is compared to the whole. A pie chart can show distribution of infection control resources.

Coordinating and conducting investigations of clusters of infection

Coordination and conduct of investigations of clusters or other adverse events should be established as part of the surveillance plan so that any adverse events trigger a chain of actions that may include the following:
- Immediate report to the infectious disease professional/committee
- Development of profile and definition of the outbreak with pertinent information, such as place, time, and/or incubation period.
- Statistical analysis of data to determine probability that adverse events occurred by chance.
- Additional laboratory specimens obtained or retesting done on existing specimens. May include targeted cultures or serologic testing.
- Review of medical records.
- Contact staff, patients, physicians and public health officials as appropriate.
- Identification of index case.
- Review of the infection control process through interviews, review of written policies and direct observation of staff procedures.
- ssessment of source of infection and development of hypothesis with case control or cohort study.
- Notification of administration or management.

Epidemiologic studies

Case control and cohort studies
Case control studies compare those with infection (cases) to a group (controls) without infection to determine if the infected group has characteristics that are different from the control group. Case control studies are done retrospectively backward from onset of infection to admission. Usually 2- 4 controls per case are assessed although the larger the number, the more significant the results. Controls should be chosen at random from the same source population of the cases. Case control studies are relatively inexpensive and can quickly assess risk factors during a possible outbreak, such as *potential* cause and effect; however, case control studies do not prove causality because there can be confounding variables. While case control studies cannot indicate relative risk, they can be used to calculate the odds ratio, that is the *estimate* of relative risk. Risk factors indicated by case control studies should be studied more conclusively.

Cohort studies
A cohort study involves a group that is studied over time. There are a number of subtypes. *Prospective cohort studies* choose a group of patients without disease, assess risk factors, and then follow the group over time to determine (prospect for) which ones develop disease. This is typical of general surveillance studies for surgical site infections. Cohort studies take more time but are more reliable statistically than case control studies. In another cohort study, an exposed group and a non-exposed group may be followed to determine how many develop a particular disease. Results are often demonstrated in "2 x 2" tables that show presence of disease and exposure/risk.

	Disease	No disease	Totals
Exposure	12	28	40
Noexposure	2	58	60
Totals	4	84	100

Data is used to calculate relative risk, or risk ratios. Retrospective cohort studies are initiated after infection develops and data is collected retrospectively from medical records to evaluate whether members of the cohort selected had exposure and developed disease.

Cross-sectional studies

A cross-sectional study assesses both disease and exposure at the same time in a target population, evaluating the presence of disease at a point in time. For example, a group of people with infections may be assessed for a particular type of exposure or exposures to determine if the exposure(s) are the cause of the infection. Cross-sectional studies can evaluate the effect of multiple variables and how they relate. Cross-sectional studies can be constructed and analyzed similarly to case control when sampling involves cases and a random selection of controls, yielding prevalence odds ratio.

If constructed as a cohort cross-sectional study with an entire group being studied at one time, a 2 x 2 table can be used and calculations would provide a prevalence ratio. Cross-sectional studies often look for the same types of data as cohort studies but require less time and are less expensive.

Comparing results to published data or other benchmarks

Comparisons to published data are always problematical and should be utilized only for guidance in establishing priorities, but there are so many variables possible from one institution to another that comparisons may not be valid. The CDC/ NNIS and now NHSN have developed benchmarks related to hospital-acquired infections based on surveillance reports of participating institutions, and these may be used for reference. Overall nosocomial infection rates should not be used for comparisons but rather risk-adjusted data for target populations because the more narrow the data, the more likely that a comparison will yield valuable information. Benchmarks that were developed as part of the baseline data for an individual institution may be a more useful source for comparison for that institution than external benchmarks because of inherent differences in populations. Additionally, staff can more easily relate to data reflecting changes within their own units and variables/risk factors can be more readily identified.

Outbreak Investigation

Preparation

Outbreak investigations may vary somewhat according to the type of outbreak, the population, and the facility, so there is no one method that will suffice for every occasion. *Preparation* includes establishment of an infection team, educating staff, assembling materials, maintaining telephone, email and other contact lists, and instituting an effective surveillance system to allow early detection of outbreaks. Outbreak investigations will include most or all of the following *steps*, but they will not necessarily be done in this order. In fact, some steps will be done simultaneously. The steps are:
- Confirm outbreak.
- Communicate regularly.
- Institute initial control measures.

- Verify diagnosis/infective agent.
- Create case definition.
- Conduct case finding.
- Investigate environment.
- Characterize cases with descriptive epidemiology.
- Develop hypotheses.
- Test hypotheses.
- Analyze data.
- Institute additional control measures.
- Evaluate control measures.
- Disseminate reports.

Confirming an outbreak

Confirming an outbreak usually begins with comparing initial outbreak data with baseline data that has been established for the institution and forming a ratio of outbreak to baseline figures. The infection control professional (ICP) should review laboratory findings of the past few weeks or months to look for trends or patterns and review medical records to look for other cases with similar diagnosis, laboratory reports, or symptoms that are suggestive of an outbreak. The initial report should be reviewed for completeness and accuracy. The target population should be reviewed for increases or changes in characteristics that might account for the apparent outbreak. If identification of the outbreak was triggered by laboratory findings, changes in laboratory procedures or increased testing or reporting could create the appearance of an outbreak. Molecular epidemiology may be initiated to create a DNA profile to determine if isolates originated from the same source.

Importance of communication

Communication is a critical issue in outbreak investigation because much information needs to be collected and disseminated. Team members should be notified of the potential outbreak so that they can begin assisting with the investigation, according to their role in the team. All physicians, managers, administrators, and staff that may be involved should be notified immediately and updated frequently as well as asked to assist in reporting new incidences of infection. The laboratory should be contacted very early as further testing may be needed and laboratory staff can provide necessary information about laboratory procedures. Laboratory staff may also be alerted to save specimens for further testing. In some cases, ancillary staff, such as housekeepers or food workers, may need to be notified as well. Depending upon the type of infection, city, county, state, or federal officials may need to be notified of an outbreak.

Initial control orders

Initial control orders may be issued as sometimes confirmation is delayed because of a need for laboratory or record review of further testing, but if an outbreak is probable and any risk is posed to others, then control orders, sometimes as simple as requiring review of handwashing procedures or placing a patient in isolation according to the type of infection, may decrease the spread of an infection.

Verifying the diagnosis/infective agent

Verifying the diagnosis/infective agent should include research about the infective agent and disease to verify symptoms and determine if characteristics of the disease are consistent with the literature. A complete clinical evaluation should be completed during this phase of the outbreak investigation. Dates and sites of cultures should be verified. Laboratory testing may be completed to verify the type of organism/isolate. DNA fingerprinting may be done as well to determine if multiple infections developed from the same source.

Case definition

The case definition defines the characteristics of a typical case in the outbreak. It serves as a guide in identifying new case:
- *Time:* The date of onset of symptoms, incubation times, and need for isolation should be noted
- *Place:* Sometimes place may extend to an entire state or be limited to a particular unit or room of the hospital.
- *Person:* Characteristics about the person could include sex, age, or general condition. If all infected patients were in the neonatal unit, then the person would be characterized as an infant.
- *Clinical presentation:* Specific symptoms or parameters for the disease should be outlined, including transmission. This may include such details as fever, rash, shortness of breath, cough, or purulent discharge.
- *Epidemiology:* This might include travel history, contact with other infected patients or staff.
- *Laboratory findings:* This should specify the type of culture results or other lab findings that would verify the infection.

Case finding

Case finding involves active steps to identify further cases of infection. Recent surveillance data should be reviewed and the laboratory notified to review lab records for indications of infection. Further testing may be ordered to identify cases. Surveillance should be increased in the areas that are affected with requests to physicians and staff to report any suspected new cases. Contact should be made with other medical providers, hospital units, or the public health department to determine if other cases have been identified especially if the original infection may have originated outside of the hospital and then spread by contact. Medical records should be reviewed carefully for symptoms or changes in condition that may warrant concern. Interviews should be conducted with those in contact with the infected patient(s) or the identified site/source of infection, and they may be referred for serologic testing or cultures.

Investigating the environment

Investigation of the environment will vary according to the type of infection and the mode of transmission. An airborne infective agent would be investigated differently than one transmitted in liquids or through feces. However, the goal of the investigation is to determine what factors in the environment have contributed to the spread of the disease:
- *Equipment* should be cultured and reuse of single-use items noted. Cleaning/use procedures should be observed. Sharing of equipment, such as blood pressure cuffs or sterilized endoscopes, should be traced by staff and patients.
- *Ventilation systems* should be checked and cultured, including air vents and filters. Records of filter changes should be verified. Air conditioning and heating units should be checked as well, especially any parts that might accumulate moisture.
- *Rooms* implicated, such as operating rooms or patient areas, must be cultured and examined carefully with cleaning procedures observed and verified. Out of hospital environmental testing may be needed.

Providing an epidemiologic description

Epidemiologic descriptions include line listings and epidemic curves.

- *Line listing* is a two-column list with variables in one column and the number and percentage of those who match that variable in the other column. Line listings can give valuable information about possible transmission or other variables. For example, a line listing of 28 cases might begin like this:

Male	21 (75%)
Smoker	7 (25%)
Clinic visit	14 (50%)
Surgery Rm. A	28 (100%)
HIV positive	21 (75%)

- *Epidemic curve* is a line or bar graph that shows the characteristics of the infection over time. Line graphs show the incidence of infection compared to baseline data. Bar graphs with time on the horizontal axis and infections on the vertical are called epidemic or epi curves and are used to plot the type of outbreak and can indicate incubation periods. Source infections often show peaks with breaks between infections but person-to-person transmission is often continuous with few peaks.

Developing and testing hypotheses

A hypothesis should be generated about the probable cause of the disease/infection based on the information available in laboratory and medical records, epidemiologic study, literature review, and expert opinion. A hypothesis should include the infective agent, the likely source, and the mode of transmission: "Surgical site infections with Staphylococcus aureus" were caused by reuse and inadequate sterilization of single-use irrigation syringes used during the operations in surgery room A." Hypothesis testing includes data analysis, laboratory findings, and outcomes of environmental testing. It usually includes case control studies, with 2-4 controls picked for each case of infection. They may be matched according to age, sex, or other characteristics, but they are not infected at the time they are picked for the study. Cohort studies, whose controls are picked based on having or lacking exposure, may also be instituted. If the hypothesis cannot be supported, then a new hypothesis or different testing methods may be necessary.

Instituting and evaluating control methods

Control methods will depend upon the hypothesis generated as to the infective agent, the source, and the mode of transmission. Control methods could include the following:

- Education of staff regarding infection control, handwashing procedures.
- Isolation of patients as appropriate, according to diagnosis.
- Serologic testing of contacts, including patients, visitors, and healthcare workers.
- Immunization as needed.
- Prophylactic antimicrobials, especially preoperatively.
- Monitoring of antimicrobials.
- Change in sterilization procedures.
- Environmental modifications.
- Reassignment of staff.
- Changes in housekeeping procedures.
- Establishment of new policies and procedures.

Evaluation of control methods is an ongoing process that begins with the initial control methods. Surveillance should continue after all control methods have been instituted and should be of sufficient duration to track changes. If there is no decrease in the number of infections, then further investigation and control methods may be necessary.

Issuing final reports

The final report is issued to all interested parties in the facility as well as public health officials and government agencies, such as the CDC, as indicated. Preparations for the final report should begin as soon as an outbreak is identified because every step of the investigation and the findings should be outlined in the report so that it serves not only as information about this one particular outbreak but can serve as a guide for future outbreaks or a recurrence. The report should include laboratory findings, line listing, and epidemiologic curves as well as procedures and results from any case control and/or cohort studies, including selection methods for control subjects. All control methods should be outlined as well as evaluation of the goals of the control methods. Questionnaires that were used to elicit information should be included in the report in the appendix so that they can be used for reference.

Infection Prevention and Control

Infection control policies and procedures

Infection control policies and procedures should be developed in accordance to CDC and accreditation standards and should be a comprehensive document that outlines administrative policies, infection control measures, and employee health measures. The infection control professional and other infection control members should be listed as well as contact information. The infection control policies and procedure manual should include policies and procedures for:

- Waste management.
- Sample forms for record keeping and reporting.
- Standard precautions and transmission-based precautions.
- Barrier protection.
- Disposal of sharps.
- Invasive devices.
- Durable medical equipment.
- Sterilization and disinfection.
- Laboratory specimens
- Patient transportation.
- Nutritional services.
- Environmental services.
- Laboratory specimens.
- Patient placement.
- Linen and laundry.
- Outpatient services.
- In-patient units.
- Recall of contaminated equipment and supplies.
- Specialized units, such as ICU, HRN, transplant units.
- Outbreak investigation.
- Serologic testing and immunization.
- Air and water quality.

Review of infection control policies and procedures should be done in response to surveillance reports, as policies and procedures should be written with clear goals and outcomes in mind. A comprehensive review should include:

- Analysis of achievement of goals: If goals are met or exceeded, then new goals may need to be set. If goals are not met, then goals may have been unrealistic or policies and procedures or training may not be adequate.
- Analysis of variances and/or outbreaks, assessing risk factors. Patterns of infection or outbreaks may indicate breakdown in the system of infection control.
- Staff input:
  - Cross-sectional questionnaires regarding compliance, knowledge, and training.
  - Meetings to discuss adequacy or problems with current policies and procedures.
- Training review: Training should be ongoing and coupled with clear expectations that staff compliance with standard precautions, including hand-washing and hand sanitation, will be 100%.

Infection control strategies

<u>Hand hygiene</u>
Handwashing
All patients are considered potentially infectious, so handwashing must be done before and after every direct contact with a patient or when removing gloves. Contamination of the hands is one of the most common causes of person-to-person transmission of infection and all medical personnel must be trained in handwashing techniques and observed regularly for compliance:
- Handwashing is done under running water with plain soap rather than antimicrobial soap because of issues related to resistance.
- Hands must be lathered thoroughly, covering all areas of the hands and wrists with soap, and then rinsed.
- After handwashing, care should be taken to avoid contact with surfaces that might serve as vectors, such as faucet handles and doorknobs.
- The faucet should be turned off by using the elbow or upper forearm or holding a piece of paper towel as a barrier.
- Hands should be dried using disposable towels.

Hand disinfection
While soap and water handwashing has been the standard for many years, in fact studies have proven that alcohol-based rubs kill twice as much bacteria in the same amount of time. They are waterless and act quickly to kill bacteria and are less irritating to the hands than repeated washing.

Hand disinfection is done for at least 15 seconds by using an alcohol-based rub, such as Purell®, and should be done before and after contact with a patient or after removal of gloves. All hand surfaces should be thoroughly coated with the alcohol-rub, including between the fingers, the wrists, and under the nails, and then the hands rubbed together until the solution evaporates. Hands should not be rinsed. Alcohol-based rubs disinfect but do not mechanically clean hands, so hands that are dirty or contaminated should be washed first with soap and water.

<u>Cleaning</u>
Cleaning involves mechanical removal of contaminants and includes both pre-cleaning and cleaning. Disinfection and sterilization procedures should be preceded by cleaning in order for them to be effective because many chemicals deactivate in the presence of organic or inorganic materials:
- Pre-cleaning includes wiping down of equipment with disposable cloths, usually dampened with detergent solution, to remove secretions, dirt, and debris. Parts should be detached so that cleaning materials can reach all surfaces. Tubes and syringes should be flushed with air or solution. Pre-cleaning should be done as quickly as possible after use to prevent an increase in microbial count.
- Cleaning includes washing with detergents or enzyme solutions (used for organic material because they promote protein lysis), often involving soaking for prescribed periods of time. Ultrasonic cleaning, which uses high-energy sound waves to dislodge debris, may be used for instruments that are difficult to mechanically clean.

<u>Disinfectants</u>
Part of infection control is to identify those items and materials that should be sterilized or disinfected as well as the type of disinfectant. There are 3 basic levels of disinfectants:
- *High* kills almost all bacteria, viruses, and fungi except for large concentrations of bacterial spores and includes hydrogen peroxide and glutaraldehyde.

- *Intermediate* kills or inactivates most vegetative bacteria (including *Mycobacterium tuberculosis),* viruses*) (HIV,* and HBV*)*, and fungi but not bacterial spores and includes sodium hypochlorite, alcohols, phenolics, and iodophors.
- *Low* kills most bacteria but only some viruses and fungi and is not effective against resistive strains or bacterial spores and includes quaternary ammonium compounds, phenolics and iodophors.

In order to meet OSHA's standards for prevention of spread of bloodborne pathogens, at least Intermediate level disinfection should be used throughout the hospital when possible, especially in labs, emergency departments, and surgery. The Environmental Protection Agency (EPA) publishes lists of registered disinfectants for different levels of disinfection.

Spalding criteria
Earle H. Spalding developed a 3-category classification system for different levels of sterilization/disinfection based on the type of item (instrument and/or equipment) and its use. While not applicable in all situations, this system is often used for reference:
- *Critical* are items or pieces of equipment entering the vascular system or sterile tissue, including breaching the mucosal barrier. These include surgical instruments, probes, and urinary catheters and must be sterilized before use. Many of these items are purchased as sterilized; others are sterilized with steam sterilization or high-level chemical sterilants, such as 7.5% stabilized hydrogen peroxide.
- *Semicritical* are those items that contact mucous membranes or non-intact skin, including respiratory and anesthesia equipments and manometry probes and catheters. These devices require high-level disinfectants, such as glutaraldehyde and hydrogen peroxide, in accordance with FDA guidelines.
- *Noncritical* are those items that come in contact with skin that is intact, such as bedpans and blood pressure cuffs. These devices require low-level disinfectants, such as alcohol or diluted bleach.

Limitations
A wide range of disinfectants must be used in a hospital because different ones have specific purposes and they are not interchangeable. Mechanical cleaning should precede disinfection. Some disinfectants have toxic fumes, some degrade materials, some are irritating to skin, so there are many considerations when choosing the correct disinfectant.

High-level disinfectants include those that are sporicidal, such as glutaraldehyde and hydrogen peroxide, but aren't used on housekeeping surfaces. These chemical sterilants are often deactivated by organic and inorganic materials, and guidelines for time, temperature, concentration, and use must be followed precisely.

Intermediate level and low level disinfectants include alcohol, which is a good general-purpose disinfectant that is compatible with other disinfectants. Iodophors are unstable at high temperatures. Chorine compounds (bleach) are effective against blood or body fluids but deteriorate rapidly when stored and are corrosive of many surfaces. Phenolics deteriorate rubber, are irritating to skin and eyes, and cannot be used on food surfaces.

Surface and air disinfection
Surface and air disinfection have been a matter of debate among healthcare providers because of costs, toxicity, and the possibility of increasing antimicrobial resistance. Studies have indicated that there is little difference in hospital-acquired infection rates with detergent use for noncritical surfaces as

opposed to disinfectant use. Noncritical surfaces are those that come in contact with intact skin and contribute minimally to infections, such as floors and walls. Some surfaces, such as bedside tables, may potentially become contaminated with blood or body fluids and should be disinfected. Some argue that floors should be disinfected because they can become contaminated and in turn contaminate detergent solutions used to clean; however, studies have shown that bacterial counts return to pre-disinfection rates within a few hours. Detergent solutions can become contaminated, but the trend toward use of pre-moistened disposable mop heads rather than bucket solutions reduces this concern. Air disinfection with aerosols is not recommended in the United States.

Sterilization

Sterilization is a process that completely destroys microorganisms, including spores. Sterilization may be done physically by different methods, including steam pressure, dry heat or ethylene oxide gas. Chemical sterilants, registered by the FDA may be used, but manufacturer's directions must be followed. In some cases, the difference between chemical sterilization and disinfection relates to the length of time the process takes. For example, many chemicals require 10-20 minutes (and some up to 12 hours) for effectiveness, but this may be impractical for cleaning of surfaces, such as floors. Sterilization can be influenced by a number of factors:

- Pre-sterilization cleaning may be inadequate, resulting in proteins or other debris that interfere with sterilizing.
- Packaging may prevent adequate contact of sterilizing agent with item.
- Loading of sterilizer must be done properly to ensure contact of sterilizing agent with all items.
- Time and temperature of sterilizer must be sufficient to kill organisms.

Reuse of single-use devices

Single use devices (SUD), such as surgical drills, catheters, and endotracheal tubes, are manufactured for one-time use, but the reality is that for many years SUDs were reused with little regulatory oversight regarding methods of disinfecting/sterilization to determine if the SUDs were safe for use. Many hospitals reprocessed their own devices although some sent them to third-party reprocessors. In response to concerns about this practice, the Medical User Fee and Modernization Act (MDUFMA) was issued in 2002, with requirements for reprocessing, including applications for 510(k)s and validation data demonstrating that the reprocessed SUD is essentially equivalent to the original SUD. Reprocessed devices are classified as critical (in contact with sterile tissue), semi-critical (in contact with mucous membranes), or non-critical (topical contact with skin only). The process of validation includes procedures for cleaning and sterilization, the types of materials, and product testing. Studies have shown that properly reprocessed SUDs are equivalent in safety to the original.

Sterilization

There are a number of different heat sterilization processes:

- *Steam* under pressure (autoclave) is the most common sterilization process, can destroy resistant bacterial spores, and can be used on most materials that are heat and moisture resistant.
- *Flash* procedures use temperatures of 132°C for 3-10 minutes, depending on whether material is porous, and kill most vegetative cells and viruses if materials are properly cleaned. It is used for surgical items that need to be quickly available for reuse.
- *Dry heat* methods are essentially hot air ovens but processing time is long. It is used for items that cannot be sterilized with steam.

Gas sterilization methods have been developed because many of the synthetic materials in use are not heat tolerant; however, many gases are highly toxic.

- *Ethylene oxide* is an effective sterilizer but is toxic and combustible, so specialized equipment is necessary to ensure safety.
- *Hydrogen peroxide plasma gas* provides low temperature, low moisture sterilization of medical devices.

Hydrogen peroxide plasma gas method
Many of the new materials in use in surgical and medical devices are damaged with heat and moisture, so alternative methods of sterilization have developed. One method commonly used is hydrogen peroxide plasma gas sterilization. Because there is no heat involved in the process, the items can be removed as soon as the process completes. There are 5 stages to the sterilization process.
1. *Chamber evacuation* creates a vacuum with reduced internal pressure.
2. *Peroxide injection* into the chamber causes the solution to evaporate and disperse throughout the chamber, killing bacteria on contact.
3. *Diffusion* of peroxide throughout chamber sterilizes items and then chamber pressure is reduced.
4. *Electromagnetic field* breaks apart peroxide vapor and creates a low-temperature plasma cloud, producing ultraviolet light and free radicals. Components then recombine into oxygen and water. Stages 1-3 repeat.
5. *Venting of chamber* equalizes pressure so chamber will open.

Variances identified through surveillance

Initial planning can facilitate responding to variances identified through surveillance. As part of the infection control plan:
- Activities should be classified according to the risk of exposure, including the need for barrier protection.
- Standard procedures should be established for all activities that might involve exposure.
- Training and education should be provided for all staff, with focus on standard precautions and handwashing.
- Compliance should be monitored on a regular basis, including monitoring of environmental surfaces.

Once a variance is identified, the framework that is already in place is used to help identify the organism and mode of transmission. Targeted infection control procedures, such as increased cleaning or disinfecting, may be indicated. Plans should already be in place for dealing with different types of organisms and modes of transmission, so an outbreak of *Clostridium difficile,* for example, would trigger a predetermined initial response, which may be varied according to the circumstances.

Specific inpatient care settings

Obstetrics
Most infections in the obstetric units are caused by migration and multiplication of the normal vaginal and cervical flora although exogenous sources are sometimes implicated. Common types of infections include:
- *Post-partum endometriosis* most-often related to Caesareans or prolonged difficult vaginal deliveries with rupture of membranes. The infection may spread and can develop into sepsis.
- *Surgical site infections, Caesarean and episiotomy,* resulting in serious infection if not promptly identified and treated. While most infective agents are endogenous, exogenous organisms, such as *Staphylococcus aureus* may be causal.
- *Urinary infections* usually related to catheterization. They are common after delivery.

- *Mastitis*, usually occurring after discharge. It is usually related to poor maternal nursing practices, such as improper care of nipples, poor feeding technique, and not emptying breasts.
- *Blood-stream infection* is uncommon and usually relates to *E.coli.* It is also associated with central venous lines.
- *Intra-amniotic infection*, most often related to rupture of membranes and prolonged labor, resulting in polymicrobial infection from normal flora.

Infection control strategies for obstetrics comprise efforts to identify and prevent infections:
- *Temperature monitoring* will identify most infections for inpatients.
- *Post-discharge* questionnaires or telephone surveys of patients and physicians can identify potential problems.
- *Preoperative shaving* should be replaced with clipping and depilatories or done immediately prior to procedures.
- *Glucose/blood sugar* control increases resistance to infection.
- *ntibiotic prophylaxis* should be with 60 minutes of incision and discontinued within 24 hours to provide protection and prevent resistance.
- *Central venous lines* using internal jugular of femoral sites should be avoided if possible or used for short periods of time. PICCs have lower infection rates. Coated catheters and use of heparin flushes may also lower chances of infection.
- *lcohol-based hand sanitizers* should be used properly before and after all patient contact.
- *Urinary catheterization* should be used only for retention as needed. Polices for catheter use and removal should be instituted.
- *Nursing/breast care instruction* should be provided to all maternal patients.

Neurology/spinal cord injuries
The most common infections in neurology/spinal cord injuries are the following:
- *Urinary tract infections* are very common and related to clean or sterile intermittent or continuous catheterization as well as urinary stasis and/or anatomic abnormalities. Infection is most often related to intestinal flora. Infections about the urethra and perineal skin are often related to condom catheter use. Bacteremia can result from severe infections.
- *Decubiti* occur in about 1/3 of patients with spinal cord injuries and are a frequent cause of infection that can invade underlying bone. Ulcers are related to pressure and contamination. Decubiti often are colonized by multiple organisms, both aerobic and anaerobic. While skin openings may be small, underlying subcutaneous and muscle tissue may be extensively compromised.
- *Respiratory tract infections*, usually pneumonia, affects about 1/3 of patients with high cervical injuries, related to invasive devices for ventilation or weakness of muscles that decreases cough reflex.

Infection control strategies for neurology/ spinal cord injuries target the most common types of infection:
- *Urinary tract infection:* Patients should be monitored for fever and/or changes in spasms or voiding habits that may indicate infection. When possible, intermittent catheterization (sterile rather than clean in the hospital) should be used rather than continuous. Antibiotic prophylaxis has not proven to be effective but bacterial interference, colonizing of the urinary tract with nonpathogenic *E. coli 83972,* has shown promising results.
- *Decubit:* Procedures for regular monitoring of skin condition, turning patients, and avoiding friction to prevent pressure from developing are critical. Both staff and patients must be

educated about prevention and skin care and cleanliness. Nutrition and hydration must be adequate to maintain integrity of the skin.

- *Respiratory infections*: Proper use of ventilation equipment must be monitored. Assisted coughing, such as through respiratory therapy and postural drainage, can reduce infections. Prophylactic antibiotics are not recommended, but patients should receive immunizations for pneumonia.

Oncology

Oncology patients are often especially at risk for both hospital-acquired and community-acquired infections because of decreased immunity, surgeries, invasive devices, and extended hospitalizations. Most infections are related to normal flora so cultures do not always identify the causative agent. Bacterial infections are the most common, followed by fungus infections and viral infections. Common infections include:

- *Respiratory tract infections* may range from rhinitis to pneumonia, occurring most commonly in patients with leukemia, lymphoma, or solid tumors involving the head, neck, or lungs.
- *Bloodstream infections* pose special risks for hematologic malignancies, but can be related to the use of tunneled central venous lines, antibiotic resistance causing an increase in Gram-positive organisms, and surgical procedures.
- *Urinary tract infections* are common and often related to catheterization.
- *Surgical site infections* are more common with extensive surgical procedures.
- *Gastrointestinal infections* may be hard to differentiate from diarrhea caused by chemotherapy, but surgery and antibiotics are risk factors.

Infection control strategies for oncology are aimed first at preventing infections:

- *Transmission-based precautions* are appropriate for some patients, especially those immunocompromised.
- *Handwashing and aseptic techniques* are especially important for person-to-person transmission.
- *Central venous line precautions* include using antimicrobial/antiseptic-coated catheters, using clear dressings that do not obscure site, and observing carefully for signs of infection.
- *Protective isolation with use of glove and gown barriers* has proven to be effective in reducing the spread of infection but is costly and not recommended for all patients.
- *Total protected environments* can be difficult to provide and expensive but may be used in selected case.
- *ir filtration* using HEPA-filtered air can be used to maintain ultra-clean air in a patient's room. The use of particulate respirators, such as the HEPA and N95 mask, by either the patient or the staff, can help to reduce inhaled pathogens.
- *Prophylactic antimicrobials and antifungals* have shown positive results but concerns about resistance developing limits use to individual cases.

Transplant patients

Infections pose a serious threat to transplant patients, especially during the first year. While opportunistic infections have decreased, nosocomial infections have increased, most related to bacterial infections. Transplant patients consistently show higher rates of infection than other patients. There are numerous potential sources:

- *Donor-infected organs* can transmit HBV, HBC, Herpesvirus, HIV, Human-T-cell leukemia virus, type I. Additionally, donors who are immunocompromised prior to harvesting of the organs may have nosocomial bacterial or fungal infections that can be transmitted. Organs can also become infected during harvesting.

- *Healthcare workers* may transmit pathogens through droplets, airborne particles, or contact, frequently transmitting pathogens on their hands or clothing.
- *lood and blood products* can transmit CMV, but transmission is rare. HCV transmission has been reduced to <1%.
- *Environmental reservoirs/sources* can include the water system, demolition activities, equipment, and surfaces. Some pathogens, such as MRSA and VRE, may be endemic to the hospital environment.

Liver transplant patients
Immunosuppression as well as the type of surgery and host responses can all be implicated as risk factors for different types of transplant patients. Liver transplant patients face a host of risk factors because long-term liver disease has often resulted in general debilitation and malnutrition.
- *Endogenous infection* of invasive candidiasis is common.
- Infections may arise from vascular and anastomotic complications.
- *Hepatic artery thrombosis* can result in gangrene and abscess formation.
- *Biliary changes* may cause blockage and stone formation, leading to infection.
- *T-tubes* inserted during surgery to maintain patency of anastomoses are prone to infections.
- *Portal vein thrombosis* may lead to infection.
- *HCV* in the host may recur, compromising the new liver and often leading to fungal infections.
- *Gastrointestinal colonization of VRE* is increasingly common in liver transplant patients, causing minor clinical difference in the host but serving as a reservoir of infection in the facility.

Kidney transplant patients
Kidney transplant patients are at risk for rejection, as are all transplant recipients, and infection.
- *Urinary catheterization* results in infection in about 50% of patients and poses a danger to the kidney if the infection spreads or becomes systemic; however, most infections, especially after 3 months, are asymptomatic and self-limiting.
- *Diabetes Mellitus* that develops shortly after transplant poses a higher risk of infection than chronic diabetes that existed prior to transplant.
- *CMV positive donor kidneys in young patients* increase the risk of serious viral infections.
- *Delayed graft function* may increase risk of bacterial infection.
- *History of chronic pyelonephritis* increases postoperative risk of infection.
- *Cadaver donor organs* are related to post-operative infection, possibly because of contamination or trauma to the organ during harvesting.
- *Preoperative hemodialysis* increases risk of bacteremia.
- *cute rejection episodes* increase risk of bacteremia.

Heart and/or lung transplant patients
Heart and/or lung transplant patients are especially susceptible to bacterial pulmonary infections, with infections occurring in 35-48% of hosts. Some risk factors place patients at increased risk:
- *CMV positive donor* places sero-negative heart and/or lung and transplant patients at increased risk for postoperative CMV pneumonia, invasive aspergillosis, and pulmonary bacterial infections.
- *Preoperative colonization of Aspergillus fumigatus* in cystic fibrosis patients poses the risk of postoperative tracheobronchial aspergillosis.
- *Colonization of resistant Pseudomonas strains* in the damaged lungs, especially in cystic fibrosis patients, can result in residual infection in other parts of the respiratory tract, providing a source of infection for the donor organs.

- *Invasive devices* such as central venous lines, circulatory assist devices, and ventilators may result in colonization and infection, especially pneumonia and sternal surgical site infections.
- *Decreased ability to cough and clear mucous* because of loss of cough reflex, pain, or weakness can contribute to pneumonia.

Pancreas transplant patients
Pancreas transplants have the highest rate of complications compared to other transplants, resulting in infection rates that range from 7-50%. Pancreas transplants may be done with (>90%) or after kidney transplants or alone for those with diabetes, type I but functioning kidneys. There are a number of factors that increase risk:
- *Underlying disease*, such as uremia and diabetes, with immunosuppression impairs healing and increases the susceptibility to infection.
- *Enteric drainage* of pancreatic enzymes into the bowel predisposes to infections by enteric bacteria.
- *Peritoneal cavity drainage* of enzymes provides a medium for pathogenic agents and increases the risk of infection and has a high rate of mortality.
- *Anastomosis* of pancreas to an internal organ may result in leakage that increases chance of infection.
- *Graft necrosis* associated with vessel thrombosis or rejection provides another medium for pathogenic agents and can result in infection.

Small bowel transplant patients
Small bowel transplants use primarily cadaveric donors to treat intestinal failure requiring parenteral nutrition to provide adequate nutrition and hydration. Small bowel transplants may be done alone or with liver or other organ transplants. About two-thirds of the patients are pediatric. However, there is significant morbidity and mortality related to the small bowel transplants with 5-year survival rates <50%. Virtually all recipients develop infection to some degree, sometimes with multiple recurrences. About 55% of deaths are caused by sepsis.
- *Intensive immunosuppression* may result in adenoviral infections of the small intestine as well as bacterial and fungal infections.
- *Cytomegalovirus or Epstein-Barr* infections caused by sero-positive donors to sero-negative recipients can lead to severe complications as large viral loads may be transmitted with the transplantation.
- *Multivisceral grafts* increase the chances of infection.
- *Bacterial translocation* may result in intra-abdominal infections and abscess formation.

Time of onset
Days 1-30: Infections that arise in the early postoperative period are often surgical site infections or other nosocomial infections.
- *cterial* infections are most common.
- *Fungal* infections, especially *Candidiasis* and *Aspergillus* usually occur early.
- *Viral* infections are less common but usually involve HSV or the herpesvirus, HHV-6.

Days 31-180: Most infections during this time period are opportunistic infections rather than nosocomial because of continued immunosuppression that increases susceptibility.
- *CMV* is the most common pathogen for all types of transplants.
- *HBV* and *HCV* may reactivate about 90 days after surgery.
- *Various pathogens* may cause infections, including *Mycobacterium tuberculosis* and *Nocardia*.

Days 181 and onward: Infections acquired after 6 months are usually community-acquired rather than hospital-acquired although the risk of opportunistic infections remains as well. Varicella zoster virus and dematiaceous fungi infections are late infections, usually after 6 months.

Viral pathogens of transplant patients
CMV
Cytomegalovirus (CMV) is the most common pathogen related to transplant infections affecting 40-90% of recipients. There are 3 types:
- *Primary infection*: seropositive organ is transplanted into a seronegative recipient, posing the most risk of rejection and other complications.
- *Reactivation infection*: latent viral infection reactivates in response to immunosuppression.
- *Superinfection:* new strain of the virus infects a seropositive recipient.

Infection control strategies may vary:
- *Serologic matching* of donor and recipients can prevent transmission; however, the limited number of seronegative transplant organs may preclude transplant surgery for many patients.
- *Early diagnosis* with the CMV antigenemia assay can yield information about the degree of infection and likelihood of CMV disease.
- *Universal antiviral prophylaxis* with ganciclovir may delay onset of CMV and decrease severity but poses the risk of increased viral resistance.
- *Targeting patients* at the highest risk for disease through surveillance methods, such as monitoring with CVM antigenemia assay and instituting prophylaxis to prevent asymptomatic disease from activating, is the most practical infection control.

HSV and VZV: Herpes simplex virus infection may occur from reactivation or primary transmission from the donor. Infection may become disseminated, most frequently affecting the liver with a high mortality rate. Infection control strategies include:
- *Serologic matching* can prevent primary transmission but the limited supply of organs may make this impractical.
- *Antiviral prophylaxis* with low dose Acyclovir (200-400 mg TID) for 1-3 months has proven very effective in preventing HSV infections.

Varicella-zoster virus infection may result in primary infection over 2 years from the time of transplant, resulting in visceral dissemination and sometimes death. This delay time may cause the symptoms to be misdiagnosed.

Infection control strategies include:
- *Immunization* has proven to be safe and highly effective, reducing the incidence of infection and the severity.
- *VZ immunoglobulin* is given to susceptible transplant patients exposed to VZV, but is not completely protective.
- *High dose acyclovir* during the 2-3 week incubation period may reduce incidence and severity of infection.

HHV-6: Human herpesvirus-6 is the newest identified viral pathogen of transplant patients, infecting 31-55% of solid organ transplants with the usual onset of symptoms (bone marrow suppression, encephalopathy, fever, and pneumonia) about 2-4 weeks after transplant. HHV-6 is a DNA virus distinct from other herpesvirus but most like CMV. There are 2 variants of the disease HHV-6A and HHV-6B. HHV-6A is more virulent than HHV-6B, but at the current time HHV-6B is the most common infection. HHV-7 is a closely related virus that often co-infects, but its significance is not yet established. Most infection with HHV-6 is endogenous from reactivation of latent virus acquired in early childhood, but primary donor transmission can also occur.

Infection control strategies include:

- *Early diagnosis* with culture assay.
- *ntiviral medications* ganciclovir and foscarnet are effective against HHV-6 infection.
- *ntiviral prophylaxis* with ganciclovir has been given BID for a week prior pre-stem cell transplant and 120 posts. Studies demonstrated a significant reduction in infection for those receiving prophylaxis.

HBV: Hepatitis B virus is a concern for both liver and kidney transplant patients because infection markedly increases mortality rates. HBV is transmitted in blood, semen, and vaginal fluids. Recurrence of HBV is most common in those already seropositive (about 83%) compared to those seronegative (about 58%) at the time of transplant, but both figures are high. Mutant varieties of HBV (precore mutants) pose an even greater threat of graft loss. HBV progresses more slowly in kidney transplant patients than in liver transplant patients, with cirrhosis and death occurring in 6-8 years compared to 2-2.5 years for liver transplant patients.

Infection control strategies include:

- *Standard precautions* should prevent bloodborne transmission.
- *Antiviral prophylaxis* with Hepatitis B Immune Globulin (HBIG) has markedly reduced recurrence rates.
- *Combination therapy* with HBIG and lamivudine prevents recurrence disease in >90% of liver transplant patients infected with HBV.
- *Hepatitis B vaccine* should be provided to adults at risk, especially staff working with patients with HBV. Children are now routinely immunized.

HCV: Hepatitis C virus causes end-stage liver disease in about half of the liver transplant patients, and 95% remain viremia after transplant, resulting in recurrence in 30-70% of patients within a year. HCV is also common in hemodialysis patients as it is a bloodborne pathogen, and 10-60% of rental transplant patents develop chronic liver disease. Co-infection with HGV occurs in about 25% without clinical impact. Most infections are reactivation, but primary transmission can occur.

Infection control strategies include:

- *Standard precautions* prevent bloodborne transmission. Up to 10% of those with needlestick injuries develop HCV.
- *Antiviral prophylaxis* using HBIG developed for hepatitis B has been shown to reduce incidence of HVC viremia because it also contains some antibodies to HCV. A new investigational Hepatitis C Immune Globulin, Civacir, is currently in trials to evaluate its prevention of recurrence of HCV infection in liver transplant patients. Civacir is made from pooled blood and serum of individuals with antibodies to HCV.

BKV: K virus (BKV) has recently emerged as a cause of renal dysfunction after transplant, resulting in loss of graft. BKV is a DNA polyomavirus, and is ubiquitous, with about 80% of the population seropositive. The transmission mode is not yet established. JC virus (JCV) often co-infects and may be a cause of nephropathy as well. About 5% of kidney transplant patients develop BKV infection (hemorrhagic and non-hemorrhagic urinary infection, nephritis, increase in creatinine, and replication of decoy cells of the urinary epithelium), usually reactivation, within 3 –24 months after surgery. Diagnosis is by PCR assay.

Infection control strategies include:

- *Reduction in immunosuppressive medications* with the addition of cidofovir (10-20% of the recommended dose of cidofovir) has been the treatment of choice with varying degrees of effectiveness.
- *Leflunomide* at immunosuppressive doses was shown in one study to eradicate BK virus. Other studies are ongoing or in progress.

AdV: Adenoviruses (AdV) comprise at least 49 serotypes and cause infections in up to 10% of pediatric transplant pediatric patients and 15% of adult, especially affecting those receiving bone marrow transplants. AdV can cause disseminated disease resulting in hemorrhagic cystitis (kidney transplants), hepatitis (liver transplants), conjunctivitis, and pneumonitis (lung transplants). AdV 11, 34, 35 are implicated in hemorrhagic cystitis while 2, 5, 7, and 9 are implicated in pulmonary infection, especially in children. Infection may be from seropositive donors or reactivation. Nosocomial outbreaks have occurred. A recent military study demonstrated serotypes 4 and 7 were transmitted through asymptomatic shedders via the respiratory tract.

Infection control strategies include:

- *Ribavarin, ganciclovir, and IgG* have been tried with varying reports as to effectiveness.
- *Vaccine* (serotypes 4 and 7) was available to the military from the 1970s to 1990s and was successful, but the vaccine was lost. Phase I trials for a new vaccine are underway and show good results.
- *Droplet precautions* should be considered, especially with respiratory infection.

Common bacterial infections after transplant surgery
Staphylococcus aureus (MRSA) and Enterococci (VREF): Staphylococcus aureus is the most common cause of bacterial infection in liver, heart, kidney, and pancreas transplant patients with >50% of infections occurring in the ICU. Intravascular cannulas cause about 54% of MRSA infections, but nosocomial transmission occurs. While nasal colonization has been implicated in infection in liver transplant patients, using mupirocin to eradicate nasal colonization has not affected infection rates, probably because of nosocomial transmission with exogenous colonization. Isolate studies have demonstrated nosocomial cross-transmission.

Enterococci are a primary concern for liver transplant patients. Vancomycin-resistant *Enterococcus faecium* (VREF) cause 10-15% of liver failures, according to recent studies. Nosocomial transmission occurs frequently, especially with prolonged hospitalization and ICU stay. Intra-abdominal infections occur about 40 days after surgery with mortality rates of 23-50%. VREF colonization puts patients at continued risk for infection and poses a reservoir for nosocomial infections. Antibiotics have been ineffective in reducing mortality rates.

Mycobacterium tuberculosis: Mycobacterium tuberculosis in transplant patients occurs in 0.35-5% of patients, a relatively low number, but the mortality rate for those infected is 30%. About a third of those infected develop disseminated disease involving extrapulmonary sites that include the gastrointestinal tract, the urinary tract, and the central nervous system. While most M. tuberculosis infection is reactivation of latent disease, nosocomial transmission of infection has occurred, especially if patients are undiagnosed so that airborne precautions are not used. Transmission has also occurred from living and cadaveric donor organs.

Infection control strategies include:

- *Airborne precautions* for diagnosed or suspected infections.

- *Identifying infected patients/staff* includes tuberculin skin testing followed by confirming radiography.
- *Prophylaxis with Isoniazid:*
    o Tuberculin reactivity ≥ 5mm
    o Newly-converted positive tuberculin.
    o Chest-x-ray showing old active TB with no prior treatment or inadequate treatment.
    o Close contact with infected individual.
    o Seropositive TB donor organ.

Legionella: Legionella pneumonia occurs in 2-9% of solid organ recipients with *Legionella pneumophila* and *Legionella micdadei* the most common forms. Some studies have reported incidence as high as 17% in heart transplant patients. Inhalation of aerosols may transmit the disease but aspiration of the bacteria occurs more frequently. *Legionella* has been traced to potable water systems providing hospital drinking water, ice machines, and ultrasonic nebulizers. Patients may develop pneumonia with or without characteristic dense nodular areas and cavitation, pericarditis, necrotizing cellulitis, and graft rejection.

Infection control strategies include:
- *Routine annual culturing* of water supply to check for *Legionella,* especially important if there are large numbers of transplant patients.
- *Positive water culture* should result in the laboratory having diagnostic tests, such as urinary antigen, available.
- *Early diagnosis* of high-risk patients should be done by routine urinary antigen testing up to 2 times weekly.
- *Water disinfecting methods:*
    o Superheating water to 70° C and flushing distal outlets.
    o Installing copper-silver ionization units.

Nocardia: Nocardia infections occur in about 2-4% of organ transplant recipients with onset from 2-8 months after surgery with pulmonary infection common but 17-38% of those infected have central nervous system involvement, which often includes brain abscesses. Lung, heart, and intestinal transplants have the highest rates of infection. Mortality rates are high for those who are infected. *Nocardia* is found in the soil and decaying vegetation, and transmission is through inhalation. Some species are more virulent than others. Nosocomial infections have occurred in clusters in transplant units related to environmental dust. Risk factors include high dose cortisone, high levels of calcineurin inhibitors (cyclosporine and tacrolimus), and CMV infection within 6 months. Calcineurin inhibitors are commonly used for immunosuppression for kidney transplants.

Infection control strategies include:
- *Environmental monitoring*
- *Antibiotic prophylaxis* with trimethoprim-sulfa-methoxazole is effective.
- *Airborne precautions* of those infected have been recommended by some.

Common fungal infections
Aspergillus: Aspergillus infections primarily involve pneumonia and sinusitis, but 25-35% disseminate systemically, and *Aspergillus* pneumonia infections have mortality rates to 85%. *Aspergillus* is a serious fungal infection in immunocompromised transplant patients, especially lung transplant patients with 8% infection rates within 9 months of surgery. Liver transplant patients have infection rates of 1-4% but disease occurs earlier, within 2-4 weeks. Heart transplant infection rates are 1-6% with disease

within 1-2 months. Aspergillus affects renal transplants the least with <1% infection rates. Prophylaxis with antifungals has not proven to be effective.

Infection control strategies include:
- *Monitoring environment and improving air filtration* with HEPA filtration or use of laminar air flow rooms for patients at high risk.
- *Construction precautions* to prevent dust and debris from circulating in patient care areas.
- *Standard precautions*
- *High resolution CT scans* should be used for early diagnosis rather than chest x-rays so treatment with voriconizole (drug of choice) can begin.

Candidiasis: Candidiasis is the most common fungal infection in transplant patients, with the exception of heart transplants. While some infections are mild, thrush and cystitis, others are invasive and life threatening, especially with the immunocompromised patient.   Infection of all organs is about 5%, but liver and pancreas transplant patients have infection rates of 15-30%. Infection may occur in the surgical site or be disseminated, posing a serious threat to the site of anastomosis. Almost all transmission of Candida is nosocomial. Endogenous transmission is common in liver transplants, but heart and lung transplants are often infected from the donor organs. Some cases have been traced to contaminated medical equipment.

Infection control strategies include:
- *Antiviral prophylaxis* with 1-2 months of fluconazole post-transplant is used at some centers, but azole-resistant strains are appearing, and there is an associated increase in *aspergillus*, so prophylaxis may be considered for only high-risk patients.
- *Monitoring of invasive devices* to ensure that they are not contaminated with *candida.*

P*neumocystis jiroveci (*formerly *carinii): Pneumocystis jiroveci* (formerly *carinii)* was classified for many years as a Protozoan, but DNA analysis has caused it to be reclassified as a fungus, but it does not respond to antifungal treatment. The variety that causes *Pneumocystis* pneumonia, commonly referred to as PCP, has been renamed as *Pneumocystis jiroveci.* While most infection is thought to be endogenous, there is sufficient evidence that person-to-person transmission has occurred in nosocomial outbreaks affecting transplant patients in contact with PCP infected HIV patients. While renal, heart, and liver transplant patients are vulnerable to *Pneumocystis,* without prophylaxis 80% of lung transplants become infected, with infection usually occurring 4 months after surgery although the length of time varies depending upon the degree of immunosuppression.

Infection control strategies include:
- *Transmission precautions* to separate PCP-infected patients from contact with transplant patients.
- *Prophylaxis* with trimethoprim-sulfa-meth oxazole should be given to all transplant patients. There is no consensus on the length of prophylaxis with durations varying from 6-12 months to indefinite.

Burn infection criteria
Burn wound cellulitis
Burn patients are at exceptional risk for infection because the barrier of protective skin is breached, eschar provides a medium for microorganisms, and immunosuppression occurs. Classifying burn infections can be done in different ways. NNIS/CDC proposed a classification system for unexcised burns, but with early excision this system often does not apply. A newer system classifies burn

infections by 4 types: cellulitis, invasive infection in unexcised burns, impetigo, and open burn-related surgical wound infection.

Burn wound cellulitis is characterized by erythema of uninjured tissue around burns that is more than the usual irritation and includes one of the following:
- Pain, tenderness and edema.
- Systemic signs of infection.
- Progressive erythema and edema.
- Lymphangitis/lymphadenitis.

This type of infection usually suggests a need for different antimicrobial treatment. When the erythema spreads beyond 1-2 cm from the burn, it may be indicative of infection with β-hemolytic *Streptococcus*.

Invasive infection in unexcised burns

Invasive infection in unexcised burns occurs when microorganisms invade partial or full thickness burns, causing a change in the appearance of the burn as well as separation and/or dark discoloration of the eschar. Other evidence of infection may include:
- Inflammation of surrounding tissue
- Biopsy indicating invasion of microorganisms into adjacent uninjured tissue
- Blood culture isolating organisms.
- Signs of systemic infection, such as hypotension, leukocytosis, hypothermia or hyperthermia.

The systemic response to a severe burn can be similar to that of an invasive infection, so careful observation of the wound and biopsy should be done because mortality rates increase markedly when the organism invades the blood stream. *Staphylococcus aureus*, *Pseudomonas aeruginosa*, Enterococci, *Enterobacter* spp. and *Escherichia coli* are the most frequent causes of infection. Since the frequent use of antimicrobials with burn patients, there has been a subsequent increase in the number of *Aspergillus* fungal infections.

Burn wound impetigo

Burn wound impetigo is an infection of previously healing and re-epithelialized partial-thickness burns, skin grafts, or donor sites. One important criterion for burn wound impetigo is that the deterioration is not caused by mechanical disruption of the tissue or by a failure to completely excise the wound but by an invading organism. Burn wound impetigo can occur with or without indications of systemic infection, such as temperature >38.4°C, leukocytosis, and/or thrombocytopenia, may be present as well. The wound may develop multiple small superficial abscesses that infect and erode the tissue. The most common cause of burn wound impetigo is *Staphylococcus aureus*. Prompt debridement of the abscesses, cleansing of the area, and application of topical antimicrobials, such as Bactroban®, must be done in order to stop the spread of the infection. A change in antimicrobial treatment may be necessary as well.

Open burn-related surgical wound infection

Open burn-related surgical wound infection usually involves an invasive infection of the excised burn site, grafts, or donor sites, and the invasive organisms are similar to those of unexcised wounds, with *Staphylococcus aureus* and *Aspergillus* frequent causative agents. The wound presents with culture-positive purulent exudate and includes at least one of the following:
- Loss of graft, synthetic or biologic.
- Change in wound appearance.
- Erythema around the periphery of the burn wound in adjacent tissue.
- Systemic signs of infections, such as temperature 38.4°C, leukocytosis, and/or thrombocytopenia.

Surface colonization by organisms in the wound may not be the same as the invading agent, so wound biopsy may be necessary. For example, *Candida albicans* frequently colonizes but rarely invades unless the immune system is severely depressed, often an impending sign of death. Changes of antimicrobial treatment as well as topical treatments are usually indicated for open burn-related surgical wound infections.

Reservoirs for organisms that infect burns
There are a number of reservoirs for organisms that infect burns. Many of these reservoirs can serve as sources for transmission on the hands of healthcare workers:
- *Burn wounds* are colonized within the first few hours by Gram-positive organisms from sweat glands and hair follicles and within days by Gram-negative organisms, so collectively the burn wounds of all patients on the unit may harbor organisms that can spread from one patient to another.
- *Gastrointestinal tract flora* can contaminate burn wounds directly if wounds are in proximity to fecal material or indirectly through cross contamination.
- *Normal flora*, especially Gram-positive cocci, on the skin are the cause of early burn infections and an increasingly important reservoir, with nasal colonization often implicated in burn infections.
- *Environment* can harbor organisms on many inanimate surfaces. Hydrotherapy equipment has been a frequent cause of wound infection as contaminated equipment spreads the infection to subsequent patients being treated.

Strategies for prevention and control
Strategies for preventing and controlling transmission of infection in burn units include the following:
- *Handwashing and sanitizing* before and after every patient contact.
- *Barriers* such as gloves and water-impermeable aprons or gowns to reduce contact transmission.
- *Environmental controls* include providing patients with individual equipment, such as stethoscopes and blood pressure cuffs, and thorough cleaning and disinfecting of all surfaces. Mattress covers should be checked. Gloves should be worn to use computers and keyboard covers cleaned daily.
- *Raw fruits and vegetables* should not be fed to patients or allowed to contaminate kitchen utensils.
- *Surveillance of all burn patients* that might serve as reservoirs of infection, including convalescent patients no longer in acute care.
- *Use of topical antimicrobials,* such as silver sulfadiazine, to control infection, but with testing of outbreak strains for resistance.
- *Protocol for systemic antimicrobial* to treat active infection but avoid development of resistance.
- *Early wound excision and closure* to reduce wound infection.

Hydrotherapy: Hydrotherapy *has* been used in burn treatment but implicated in a number of nosocomial outbreaks, primarily of *Pseudomonas aeruginosa*. In some cases, rigorous cleaning protocols have reduced infection; in others, suspension of hydrotherapy treatments was needed. Because of problems with infection, there has been decrease in the use of hydrotherapy. Methods to control transmission of infection include:
- *Protocol* for draining tub after use and cleaning and disinfecting all parts of the hydrotherapy tub and agitators, with a chlorine germicidal agent circulated through agitators. Tank to be rinsed and dried thoroughly.
- *Environmental* cleaning and disinfecting of complete area and transportation equipment.

- *Disinfectant* may be added to filled tank.
- *Disposable plastic liners*, shown to reduce but not eliminate infection.
- *Barriers* such as long gloves and aprons or gowns impervious to fluid to prevent contact with water or patient.
- *Faucets* without stream diverters or aerators, which might harbor organisms, flushed with hot and cold water before use.

Respiratory therapy
Strategies for prevention and control
Respiratory equipment has been implicated as the cause of many nosocomial infections, so preventing and controlling transmission of infection during respiratory therapy is imperative. Control measures include:
- *Specific procedures* for different types of respiratory equipment/procedures.
- *Standard precautions* at all times.
- *Cleaning* all equipment prior to disinfecting/sterilizing.
- *Disinfect*ing/sterilizing all equipment as directed by manufacturer, with steam sterilization or high-level disinfection.
- *Disposable* equipment used by only one patient and changed as directed by manufacturer.
- *Scheduled draining* of condensate in ventilator/other tubing.
- *Using closed-continuous feed humidification* system/ heat-moisture exchange (HME).
- *HME* changed daily.
- *Single-dose sterile medications* used at all time.
- *Sterile/pasteurized* nebulizer fluid administered aseptically.
- *Avoiding intubation* when possible.
- *Avoid high-volume humidifiers* unless sterilized daily and used with sterile water.
- *Nursing* practices aimed at reducing pneumonia (turning, kinetic beds, elevating head of bed, deep breathing and coughing exercises)

Operating rooms
Strategies for preventing and controlling transmission of infection in operating rooms includes:
- *Preoperative surgical scrubs* for 3-5 minutes and aseptic techniques at all times.
- *Positive-pressure ventilation* with respect to corridors and adjacent areas.
- *≥15 air exchanges per hour (ACH)* with at least 3 fresh air.
- *Filtering* of all recirculated and fresh air though filters with 90% efficiency.
- *Horizontal laminar airflow* or introduction of air at ceiling and exhaust near the floor level.
- *Operating room closed* except to allow passage of essential equipment and staff.
- *Clean visible soiling* with approved disinfectants between patients.
- *Wet-vacuum* operating room at end of each day.
- *Sterilize surgical equipment* and avoid use of flash sterilization.
- *Perform environmental sampling* of surfaces or air as part of epidemiological investigation.
- *Establish protocols for patients with airborne precautions,* such as tuberculosis.

Support services

Housekeeping
Strategies for preventing and controlling transmission of infection in environmental services in housekeeping are important because VRE and *Aspergillus* infections have been linked to environmental sources. Daily cleaning strategies include:
- *Gloves* for all cleaning.

- *Damp-mopping all floors*, with disposable mop cloths if possible.
- *Waste baskets* emptied and re-lined with plastic bags.
- *Horizontal surfaces,* such as bedside stands, cleaned with a disinfectant solution approved by the EPA.
- *Bathrooms* thoroughly cleaned, including vector-surfaces, such as faucet handles and doorknobs.
- *Soap* and *alcohol antiseptic* dispensers checked and refilled.
- *Barrier precautions,* such as long gloves, gowns, masks, goggles, or respirators should be used if indicated for cleaning blood or body fluids that may splash or spatter during cleaning procedures, when handling large volumes of fluids or dirty linen, or if patient on airborne precautions.
- *Terminal cleaning* includes disinfecting all parts of the bed and equipment and all room furniture, disposal of non-reusable equipment, disinfecting and/or sterilization of reusable equipment.

Linen services/laundry

Linen is frequently contaminated with blood and body fluids and serves as a source of contamination. Control strategies include:
- *Manipulating* linen as little as possible, avoiding fanning linen.
- *Gloves or other barrier precautions* worn for contact with contaminated linen or sorting.
- *Sort/rinse* linen away from patient care areas (except for rinsing fecal material from linen in dirty hopper utility room).
- *Bag* soiled linen at source location.
- *Leak-proof* linen bags in use.
- *Linen chutes* cleaned on scheduled basis and as needed.
- *Ventilation system* should preclude exchange of air from laundry to patient areas.
- *Soiled laundry area* should be separate from patient care areas and storage area for clean linen.
- *Low temperature washing* may be used with controlled amounts of bleach as per established guidelines.
- *Transportation* of clean and dirty linen must be separate.

Nutritional services

Nutritional services staff should be trained to safely deliver food to patients. Disposable dishes and silverware are not necessary for infection control.
- Nutritional services staff deliver food trays to all patients except for those on airborne precautions.
- Medical personnel deliver trays to those on airborne precautions.
- Trays must not be delivered if the over-head table is contaminated with equipment, such as a bedpan, or body fluids, such as blood. Medical staff must be notified so that they can remove the material, disinfect the table, and deliver the tray.
- Nutritional services staff pick up all trays except those on airborne precautions.
- Trays must not be picked up if they contain medical equipment (such as syringes) or are contaminated with body fluids or wastes. Medical staff must be notified so that they can resolve the issue. Non-disposable dishes or utensils contaminated with body fluids must be placed in a decontamination bag or container and taken to central supply services for reprocessing.

Diagnostic procedures and devices

Short-term intravascular devices

Strategies for reducing infection risks associated with intravascular devices include:

- *Site selection* away from the internal jugular or femoral veins, using PICC if possible.
- *Tunneled catheter or ports* used if possible because of lower infection rates than non-tunneled catheters.
- *TPN catheters* used only for TPN and not other procedures.
- *Experienced trained staff* to insert intravascular devices.
- *Dressings* may be transparent or gauze, but insertion site should be examined frequently by palpation and dressing removed for inspection on any tenderness. Change dressings at least 1 time weekly.
- *Using maximum aseptic technique* for insertion.
- *Catheter material* of Teflon® or polyurethane, which demonstrates lower rates of infection than polyvinyl chloride or polyethylene; catheters impregnated with antimicrobials have demonstrated reduction in infections.
- *Rotation of catheter sites* every 72-96 hours (for adults) for short peripheral venous catheters but only as needed for others.
- *Avoid antibiotic ointments* at insertion site because of danger of fungal infections or resistance.

Urinary catheters

Strategies for reducing infection risks associated with urinary catheters include:
- *Using aseptic technique* for both straight and indwelling catheter insertion.
- *Limiting catheter use* by establishing protocols for use, duration, and removal, training staff, issuing reminders to physicians, using straight catheterizations rather than indwelling, using ultrasound to scan the bladder, and using condom catheters.
- *Utilizing closed-drainage systems* for indwelling catheters.
- *Avoiding irrigation* unless required for diagnosis or treatment.
- *Using sampling port* for specimens rather than disconnecting catheter nd tubing.
- *Maintaining proper urinary flow* by proper positioning, securing of tubing and drainage bag, and keeping drainage bag below the level of the bladder.
- *Changing catheters* only when medically-needed.
- *Cleansing external meatal* area gently each day, manipulating the catheter as little as possible.
- *Avoid* placing catheterized patients adjacent to those infected or colonized with antibiotic-resistant bacteria to reduce cross-contamination.

Bronchoscopy

Bronchoscopy poses risks of spreading infection distally from the upper respiratory tract, transmitting infection to other patients from contaminated equipment, and transmitting infection to staff. Of primary concern are pathogens that survive and multiply in water, such as *Pseudomonas* or mycobacteria. Pseudo-epidemics may occur if scopes are environmentally contaminated as colonization may be from the scope rather than related to infection in the patient. Control strategies include:
- *Thorough mechanical cleaning* immediately after use to prevent drying of secretions.
- *Sterilization or high-level disinfection* with EPA-approved agents as directed, manually or with automated endoscopic reprocessor, with dismantling of all components of the scope to ensure proper disinfection and sufficient duration. Sterile rinses and sterile transport cases must be used to ensure that environmental contamination does not take place.
- *Monitoring of automated endoscopic reprocessor* for contamination.
- *Use of disposable* devices for parts that are difficult to adequately clean.

Angiography, angioplasty, and percutaneous trans-catheter embolization

Strategies for reducing infection risks associated with angiography, angioplasty, and percutaneous trans-catheter embolization include:

- *Using standard precautions with barrier protection,* such as gloves, gowns, and goggles, as well as strict aseptic technique with surgical drapes that are liquid resistant.
- *Avoiding shaving* when possible or using electric shaver.
- *Using antiseptic* on insertion site.
- *Antibiotic prophylaxis* in selected individual, such as the immunocompromised, or selected procedures, such as embolization.
- *Avoiding cutdown procedures,* which have higher rates of infection.
- *Removing catheters* as soon as possible.
- *Avoiding non-permeable plastic dressings* in favor of gauze or semi-permeable transparent dressings.
- *Avoiding disposing of contaminated fluids* or flushing of catheter into an open container.
- *Limiting reuse of equipment* to those allowed by federal regulations,
- *Cleaning and disinfecting* any non-disposable equipment following manufacturers' directions.
- *Environmental precautions* as per operating room.

Hemodialysis
Strategies for reducing infection risks associated with hemodialysis include CDC precautions:
- *Use standard precautions* and gloves. Wash/sanitize hands between each patient.
- *Items taken into dialysis area* should be disposed of, used on only one patient, or cleaned and disinfected prior to returning to central area for use on another patient.
- *Use single-dose medications* or multi-dose vials for one patient and do not return to central area; conversely, prepare medications from a multi-dose vial in central area and deliver separately.
- *Do not use a common medication cart* for multiple patients.
- *Maintain separate clean and contaminated areas* that are non-adjacent.
- *Use external venous and arterial pressure transducer filters/protectors* for individual patients, change between patients, and do not reuse.
- *Clean and disinfect* entire dialysis station, including all furniture and equipment (with control panels), between patients.
- *Use leak proof containers* to transport dialyzers and tubing for reprocessing according to industry standards.
- *Vaccinate susceptible patients for HBV; establish* routine testing protocol for HBV and HCV.

Latex exposure
Latex allergies related to proteins in natural latex, which is a form of sap, have caused serious reactions in both staff and patients. Increasingly, hospitals use alternative materials, such as plastic and nitrile in place of latex, but knowing which equipment and materials, such as gloves and medical stoppers or ports on IVs, contain latex is important in preventing reactions. Reactions may range from contact dermatitis and hypersensitive allergic dermatitis to anaphylaxis and death. Patient's rooms, identification bands, and charts should carry clear indication of allergies. Staff allergies may require assessment of latex in use and changes in equipment. Routes of exposure include the following:
- Contact through direct touching can result in cutaneous, mucosal, or percutaneous exposure.
- Parental exposure may be related to IVs with latex ports or injections into system with syringes containing dry latex.
- Inhalation can result from inhaling protein particles from someone in the room using powdered latex gloves.

Medical waste disposal

Medical waste management is mandated by Federal and state laws, which require that certain types of medical waste be separated from others. This regulated medical waste (RMW) is eventually packaged, transported, and disposed of according to specific regulations for the type of waste material. Separate trash containers, lined with red plastic bags or containers and labeled as "Biohazard," must be provided for RMW, which includes:

- *Sharps* include needles, syringes, small vials, pins, probes, and lancets.
- *Blood and body fluid contaminated* material that can drip fluid: sponges, specimen containers, drainage bags (such as Hemovacs), and contaminated tubing.
- *CDC Bio-safety Class 4- associated waste*, such as those related to Marburg hemorrhagic fever.
- *Laboratory materials*, including cultures, infectious agents, and contaminated materials.
- *Animal waste* related to medical research.
- *Human tissue* includes body parts removed during surgery or autopsy.
- *Chemotherapy* waste containing over 3% antineoplastic drugs.

Sharps disposal

Injuries, especially needle-sticks, related to medical instruments such as scalpels and needles (sharps), are very common but pose a serious risk of infection. Care should always be used when sharp instruments or needles, and assistance should be obtained when using sharps with people who are confused or uncooperative, increasing the chance of injury. The following guidelines should be used:

- A special sealed sharps container should be available in every room where treatment is done (patients rooms, clinics, operating rooms).
- Disposable needles should not be removed, recapped, or touched but deposited immediately into the sharps container. If recapping cannot be avoided, the scooping method of recapping using only one hand must be used.
- The sharps container must be checked daily and removed for disposal when about 3/4 full and a new container provided.
- Any non-disposable sharps must be placed in a covered container that is leak and puncture proof and returned to the central supply department for cleaning and sterilization.

Recall of potentially contaminated equipment and supplies

The FDA maintains regulates procedures and recall regarding contaminated equipment and supplies a website entitled MedWatch (http://www.fda.gov/medwatch/index.html) to provide safety information for drugs and medical equipment. MedWatch provides electronic listing service to medical professionals and facilities for the following:

- Medical product safety alerts.
- Information about drugs and devices.
- Summary of safety alerts with links to detailed information.

The Safe Medical Practices Act (1990) requires manufacturers and medical device user facilities to report problems with medical devices, including deaths or serious injuries (defined as requiring medical or surgical intervention), within 10 working days. Facilities must also file semiannual reports on January 1 and July1. User facilities must maintain records for 2 years and must develop written procedures for identification, evaluation and submission of medical device reports (MDR). MedWatch provides:

- *Reporting forms* (downloadable) for voluntary and mandatory reports

- *Recall and safety information* about recalls, market withdrawals and safety alerts, organized by months and years.

Ambulatory care centers

Ambulatory care centers comprise a wide range of facilities, from those that are within the hospital to freestanding, prison based, or physician's office surgical centers. They pose a particular challenge for the ICP, who must work with personnel and computer systems in order to collect data. Numerator and denominator data may be difficult to establish, and patient populations may vary widely. Because stay is short-term, many infections or problems may present only after discharge. Control strategies include:
- *Definitions* that allow for comparison.
- *Procedures for surveillance* and identifying staff to assist/train.
- *Targeting* particular types of infections or populations.
- *Reporting procedures* for results of surveillance.
- *Strict adherence* to standards of asepsis and care.
- *Post-discharge surveillance:* letters, telephone calls to patients and physicians.
- *Institution of outcomes* and changes based on results.
- *Standard infection control* procedures as per hospital operating rooms.*Sentinel events* such as death or impairment resulting from nosocomial infection.

Barrier/Isolation precautions

Gloves

Barrier precautions are used to prevent infection in accordance with mode of transmission and likelihood of contamination with blood or other body fluids or wastes:
- *Gloves* are worn when hands may make contact with body fluids, including mucous membranes, or instruments that have made contact with body fluids, or any skin that is not intact, such as cuts, scrapes, or chapped. Gloves should be worn to protect the patient from any cuts or other breaks in the skin of the caregiver. Sterile gloves are used for sterile procedures.

Gloves are used not only to prevent the spread of pathogenic agents from one patient to another but also to protect the healthcare worker. There are limitations to the degree to which gloves can control infections because transmission is complex. For example, gloves offer no protection to infections caused by endogenous flora.

There are a number of different types of gloves available. Traditionally nurses and surgeons have relied on latex gloves, which pose a danger to those who are allergic to latex. Now healthcare workers in almost all departments use gloves, so they must be widely available in all patient rooms and departments, so strength and versatility are important.
- *Latex* is strong, flexible and has some reseal ability, but contains proteins that cause allergic reactions.
- *Chloroprene/Neoprene* similar to latex in strength and flexibility, resists puncture, but tears more easily. It contains chemical accelerators.
- *Nitrile* is strong and resistance to tears and punctures. Less flexible than latex, it contains chemical accelerators.
- *Vinyl* is weak, inflexible, tears ad breaks easily and contains chemical accelerants.

- *Polyurethane* is durable, resistant to tears and punctures and superior to latex. It contains no proteins or chemical accelerants.
- *Copolymer* punctures easily but is resistant to tears, and is stronger than vinyl but less flexible than latex. It contains chemical accelerants.

Gowns

The CDC guidelines for barrier precautions call for the use of a clean non-sterile gown. Sterile gowns are reserved primarily for surgical procedures. There are a variety of different types of aprons and gowns that are available, primarily for the protection of the healthcare worker, but gowns also reduce contamination of uniforms and thus protect patients.

Gowns should be moisture-resistant and easily cover clothing. They are worn to prevent contamination from blood or body fluids during activities or procedures that may result in splashing or splattering. They should be changed after caring for the patient or procedures that may have resulted in contamination. Gowns should be handled as little as possible, sliding down raised arms and fastening at the neck, with gloves pulled over sleeves. Gown should be removed before gloves to reduce hand contamination, and the hands should be washed immediately after gloves are removed.

Goggles and face shields

The face is particularly vulnerable to splashing and splattering of blood and body fluids because staff are often leaning over the patients during procedures. The mucous membranes of the eyes, nose, and mouth can become contaminated, so protective eyewear and face shields should be worn when contamination of the face is possible:
- *Goggles* should be non-vented or indirectly vented with an anti-fog coating and should allow for direct and peripheral vision. They should be large enough to cover eyeglasses if necessary and still fit snugly to provide protection.
- *Face shields* provide protection to the eyes and face. The shields should have both crown and chin protection and should extend around the face to the ears. Small, thin disposable shields that attach to surgical masks provide more limited protection.

Both goggles and face shields should be washed with soap and water after each use and disinfected with 70% alcohol if contaminated.

Masks and respirators

Masks can provide protection from droplets, but they do not provide protection from smaller airborne microorganisms. Respirators that contain filters must be used for airborne precautions.
- *Masks* are used primarily to protect patients from droplets during sterile procedures, but are used when working within 3 feet of a patient on droplet precautions. They provide protection of the mucous membranes of the nose and mouth from spraying or splattering of blood or body fluids.
- *Respirators* must be used for protection against airborne transmission. The National Institute for Occupational Safety and Health (NIOSH) establishes requirements for respirators, which must filter 95% of 0.3um-sized particles in order to protect against *Mycobacterium tuberculosis.* These are referred to as N95 respirators.
- The disposable N95 can be reused if not visibly damaged or dirty with TB patients but must be disposed of after use if patients are also on contact precautions (smallpox, SARS).

Respirators that are not properly fitting will not provide adequate protection against airborne particles. Fitting must be done prior to use for anyone who will use a respirator. OSHA has established guidelines for fitting and use of respirators. The staff must be tested with the same make, model, and size of respirator they will use.

- Numerous factors can affect seal: facial hair, makeup, bone structure, scars, and dentures.
- Sensitivity testing involves placing the subject's head into a hood and then squeezing a test solution of saccharine or denatonium benzoate into the hood in increments to determine when the subject can taste the solution.
- The qualitative fit test involves wearing the respirator for 5 minutes; then, the hood is placed over it and the test solution is squeezed into the hood to determine if the respirator fits tightly enough to prevent the subject from tasting the solution.
- Exercise, such as talking, moving, bending, and jogging must be done to check security of seal.

Isolation precautions

Airborne infection isolation should be initiated with suspicion or confirmation of a diagnosis of disease that has airborne transmission, such as varicella-zoster virus (VZV), measles, variola (smallpox), and tuberculosis, with droplet size <5μm, or patients with multiple drug-resistant strains of organisms. Isolation should be continued until confirmation that patient is not infective. Isolation procedures include:

- Placing patient in a private room with $\geq$ 12 air exchanges per hour (ACH) under negative pressure with air from the outside in and exhaust, preferably, to the outdoors, or recirculation provided through high-efficiency particulate air (HEPA) filters.
- Door to the room should remain closed and sign or color/coding should be used at door to alert medical staff to isolation.
- Respirator use for personnel entering room when indicated because of disease transmission (TB and smallpox) or lack of immunity (measles, VZV).
- Patient transported in clean linens and wearing a facemask.
- Procedures done in the room whenever possible.

Special protective environment isolation

While isolation is usually intended to protect others from an infected patient, protective environments (PE) are usually used to protect a severely immunocompromised patient. Most often, protective environments are provided in specialized hospital units, such as those for stem-cell transplant. Patients who are identified by diagnosis should be placed immediately in the protective environment and maintained in the environment until immune or clinical status improves. Protective environments include:

- Placing patient in a private room (or room shared by cohort) with positive airflow from the room to the outside so that contamination from the hallway or other rooms is avoided. ACH is $\geq$ 12 and HEPA filtration is used to prevent contamination.
- Gown and gloves are used to reduce transmission of pathogens, but mask is not needed unless the patient is also on droplet precautions.
- One to one nursing should be utilized.
- Patient should leave room only if medically necessary and in clean linens with face mask if necessary and 2-person transport.

Patient Placement and Environmental Inspections

Patient placement issues

The use of standard precautions obviates most patient placement in private rooms, but private room placement is necessary under some conditions:

- *irborne transmission:* Airborne precautions must be used. Room should have negative pressure if possible.
- *Droplet transmission:* Droplet precautions must be used. Patient may share a room with another patient infected with the same microorganism if there are no other contraindications.
- *Microorganism transmitted by contact:* Contact precautions must be used. Patient may share a room with a patient colonized or infected by the same microorganism.
- *Contaminated environment:* Patients producing large amounts of body fluids or waste, such as blood or stool, that cannot be contained should be placed in a private room.
- *Poor hygiene:* Patients not willing or are too confused or unable to properly maintain hygiene should be placed in private rooms.

Private rooms should be assigned when possible by Admissions utilizing a list of specific diagnoses.

Evaluating patient care environment

Environmental inspections to evaluate infection control practices and hazards requires a multi-faceted approach that includes:

- Surveillance reports regarding the incidence of infection.
- Feedback of reports to staff.
- Observation of clinical practice.

In all facilities, environmental inspections should be ongoing, but in large facilities, observing all staff for compliance with infection control practices can be difficult if not impossible, so utilizing surveillance reports to target areas of concern may be more time and cost effective. Once an area is targeted, feedback should be provided to staff and comprehensive inspections should include direct observation of staff during clinical work rather than staff demonstrations. The ICP or designated team members should participate in the investigation. Environmental culturing may be done as well as staff cultures when indicated. Questionnaires may be used to solicit information about staff compliance, understanding of infection control, and satisfaction with training.

Air and water quality

The CDC and the Healthcare Infection Control Practices Advisory Committee (HICPAC) provide recommendations for air and water quality in healthcare facilities. While air quality is a major concern, there is little evidence of contaminated air resulting in surgical site infections although spores of *Aspergillus* in the environment have been implicated in infections. Environmental services maintain both negative and positive pressure rooms and monitors air flow and filtration. Recommendations include:

- Ensuring that heating, ventilation, and air-conditioning (HVAC) filters are installed properly and maintained without leaks or dust overloads.
- Engineering humidity controls in the HVAC system to ensure adequate moisture removal.
- Ensuring air intakes and outputs are located properly and maintained to ensure operation.
- Providing portable HEPA filter units to augment room filtration.

- Using airborne sampling tests to evaluate integrity of barriers.
- Maintaining water temperatures in the correct range (hot $\geq 51°C$ and cold $\leq 68°C$ or state requirements), with constant recirculation of hot water in patient areas.
- Testing water and water equipment for microbes.

Hospital ventilation systems

There are a number of different types of ventilation systems that are used in medical facilities. Heating, ventilation, and air conditioning (HVAC) systems must not only circulate air but also exhaust the stale air to reduce contaminants and provide filtration.
- *Central air conditioning* is relatively inexpensive but doesn't allow for separate control of temperature in different areas.
- *Dual duct system* has separate heating and cooling systems with two ducts that feed into mixers, allowing for thermostats in individual rooms.
- *Filtration* is needed in addition to other HVAC systems to remove small particles. Filters are rated for efficiency and must be changed regularly. Outdoor air is often filtered by 20-40% efficient filters, mixed with recirculating air, and then refiltered with 90% efficient filters.

Major concerns related to HVAC are that filtration is adequate, filters are changed regularly, and moisture is prevented from building up and providing a medium for microorganisms.

Positive pressure rooms

A positive pressure (protective environment) room creates a protective environment for patients who are immunocompromised. In these rooms, the pressure is positive within the room so that clean air flows out of the room to the "dirty" area of the hallways, protecting the patient from pathogens. Air exchanges are >12 per hour, and filtration is by 99.97% HEPA filters. Windows should be sealed for protection and the room outfitted with self-closing doors. Positive pressure rooms are used for those who are immunocompromised:
- HIV/AIDs patients with reduced immunity.
- Oncology patients wit bone marrow suppression.
- Solid organ transplant patients.

In the operating room
In an operating room, a positive pressure environment must be maintained with the area of the operating table and the patient considered "clean." Filtered air in large volumes washes over the table from the ceiling and then is drawn to the air returns around the margin of the room. Air displacement must assure that any pathogens shed by the operating room personnel are moved away from the patient by the force of air. Windows should remain sealed and doors closed to maintain the proper pressure and air flow. Air exchanges are 15-25 per hour and 90% filters are used. It is also very important that barriers, such as masks and gowns, be used by all staff to prevent the shedding of bacteria into the operative area and that all surfaces be clean. Local exhaust and filtration systems to capture odors or aerosols generated during operative procedures may be used in addition to the room filtration system

Laminar air flow rooms

Laminar air flow (LAF) rooms provide more protection than a positive pressure room because one entire wall is composed of HEPA filters and fans blow air at high velocity through the filters with >100 air exchanges per hour, creating drafts and noise. Staff should work "down wind" of patients, who are severely immunocompromised (such as bone marrow transplant patients).

Negative pressure rooms

Negative pressure (isolation) rooms are devised as isolation rooms to protect those outside the room from airborne pathogens. In these rooms, air flows from the outside (clean) into the room (dirty) and then to the exterior of the building so that it doesn't recirculate. If recirculation is necessary, it must be through a HEPA filter. Air exchanges are ≥ 6 in renovated rooms or > 12 in new construction. Windows must remain sealed and doors closed as much as possible to maintain negative pressure. Negative pressure rooms are more difficult to engineer than positive pressure rooms. Negative pressure rooms are used primarily for active infections with *Mycobacterium tuberculosis* (TB) causing a cough with aerosolized infectious particles. Patients who have TB and are immunocompromised, such as those co-infected with HIV pose particular problems. In some cases a positive pressure room is inside a negative pressure room. Another solution is a freestanding positive pressure facility with the air exiting through filters into the fresh air.

Control risk assessment for construction projects

Construction can release air or waterborne infective organisms into the environment, so all construction should be planned with the ICP and other team members in order to minimize contamination. Risk control includes:
- Procedures for approval of projects.
- Protocols for reducing dust and debris exposure during construction.
- Clear outline of responsibilities for supervision of all aspects of the building process to ensure compliance with safe air/ water standards.
- Plan for environmental services to clean work areas, new construction, and renovated areas as well as inspection when project completed.
- Identification of high-risk patients and relocation if necessary.
- Restriction of admission of immunocompromised patients during construction if necessary.
- Staff training regarding dangers of construction to patients.
- Evaluation of risk and environmental testing and cultures, including air sampling.
- Final inspection prior to admitting patients to new or renovated area.

Communicable diseases and special situations

Cystic fibrosis patients

Cystic fibrosis (mucoviscidosis) is a progressive congenital disease that particularly affects the pancreas and lungs causing digestive and respiratory problems. It is caused by a genetic defect that affects sodium chloride movement in cells, including mucosal cells that line the lungs, causing the production of thick mucus that clogs the lungs and provides a rich medium for bacteria. Cystic fibrosis patients usually suffer from recurrent respiratory infections of the lower respiratory tract. The most common infective agents are *Pseudomonas aeruginosa* and *Burkholderia cepacia* complex. Patients with chronic infections serve as reservoirs for patient-to-patient transmission of infection, with proximity and duration of contact as precipitating factors. Cystic fibrosis patients should be maintained on universal and droplet precautions and placed in private rooms or cohorted with someone with the same pathogen.

Tuberculosis

Tuberculosis (TB), caused by *Mycobacterium tuberculosis,* is not a new disease, but an increase in resistant strains has brought control and prevention of tuberculosis to the forefront of infectious disease control. TB is a particular danger to those who are immunocompromised, with 8-10% of those with HIV developing TB. Patients with TB may develop weight loss, general debility, night sweats, and fever. With pulmonary involvement, a progressive cough resulting in dyspnea and bloody sputum is common. Diagnosis is based on skin and sputum testing as well as x-ray. Transmission is from airborne particles small enough to suspend in the air, so anyone in contact to someone with active TB is at risk of inhaling particles.

Precautions:
- Prompt diagnosis and anti-tuberculosis drugs.
- irborne infection isolation.
- Skin testing/x-rays of those in contact.
- Preventive Isoniazid therapy for those with latent infection or newly converted to positive on TB testing.

SARS

Severe Acute Respiratory Syndrome (SARS) is caused by a corona virus (Co-V) and presents as a respiratory illness with fever, cough, dyspnea, and general malaise is extremely virulent, spreading easily from person to person through close contact by way of contaminated droplets produced by coughing or sneezing. SARS has a high mortality rate. Some possibility exists that SARS may also have airborne transmission in some cases with aerosol-producing procedures. High rates of infection have occurred in healthcare workers and others in contact with infected patients, so prompt diagnosis and proper isolation are essential.

Precautions:
- Contact and droplet precautions, including eye protection and appropriate personal protection equipment.
- Airborne precautions (recommended by the CDC), especially with aerosol-producing procedures (ventilators, nebulizers, intubation).
- Immediate notification of public health authorities and institution of contact tracing.
- Activity restrictions of exposed health care workers planned in coordination with public health officials.

Methicillin-resistant *Staphylococcus aureus* (MRSA)

Methicillin-resistant *Staphylococcus aureus* (MRSA) is caused by a mutation in *S. aureus*, causing it to be resistant to methicillin (amoxicillin) and other beta lactamase-resistant penicillins as well as cephalosporins. First identified in 1945, MRSA has become endemic in hospitals and is increasingly the cause of surgical site and bloodstream infections and pneumonia with over half of *S. aureus* infections now MRSA and mortality rates of 21%. MRSA is often colonized on the skin and especially in the anterior nares and can easily spread through contact with contaminated surfaces or hands. Community-acquired as well as hospital-acquired infections are of grave concern.

Precautions:
- Prompt diagnosis and treatment with Vancomycin or other antibiotics.

- Standard and contact precautions with use of gloves and gown. Masks may also be used, especially if patient has pneumonia.
- Droplet precautions with pneumonia.
- Place patient in private room or cohort.
- Routine surveillance of high-risk patients or those with previous history of MRSA.

Vancomycin resistant enterococci (VRE)

Vancomycin resistant *enterococci* (VRE) was first identified in 1986 but has shown a rapid increase in both intensive care units and medical/surgical units with about 25% of *enterococci* infection now VRE. Patients who are immunocompromised or severely ill are at increased risk as well as those admitted to intensive care units or hospitalized for lengthy periods. VRE is also associated with antibiotic use, including vancomycin and others, such as Clindamycin and Ciprofloxacin. VRE can occur systemically or infect the urinary tract or surgical sites. Some people are colonized but have no symptoms although they may pose a threat to others as it may survive on surfaces for up to 6 days.

Precautions:
- Isolation with barrier precautions, gown and gloves, during all patient contact, even entering room.
- Hand hygiene both before and after contact and use of gloves.
- Use of dedicated equipment to reduce transmission.
- Policy to limit vancomycin use.
- Thorough cleaning of isolation room.

Pandemic influenza

Pandemic influenza is a worldwide epidemic of influenza that causes serious respiratory illness and/or death in large populations of people. Pandemics can occur when a virus mutates, creating a new subtype that infects humans and spreads easily from person to person. The influenza of most concern recently has been avian flu, which primarily affects birds, but has infected other animals, including humans, primarily those in contact with infected flocks. There are a number of subtypes of avian flu and symptoms may range from typical influenza-like respiratory infections to severe pneumonia. Should a further mutation occur and a pandemic occur, the implications for health care are profound because of the potential number of infected patients overwhelming the medical system.

Precautions:
- Standard precautions with careful hand hygiene.
- Contact precautions with gloves and gown for all patient contact and goggles when within 3 feet.
- Dedicated equipment.
- Airborne precautions in isolated negative pressure rooms and use of N-95 filter respirator.

Products and medical equipment

Wheelchairs and walkers

Wheelchairs are ubiquitous in the healthcare facility and often are used to transport many different patients between various units in the hospital without intervening cleaning or disinfection. However, they may become contaminated with urine, feces, and food. Organisms on the hands can be easily transmitted to the arms of the chairs or walkers and then to the next occupant. Walkers, while often dedicated to one patient, pose a similar danger if used for multiple patients. Control of transmission should include:

- *Barriers for transportation*, such as a clean sheet between the patient and the wheelchair with waterproof disposable pads if necessary to protect against urine, feces, blood, or other discharge.
- *Inspection after use* should be done each time and if soiled, it should be immediately removed from service, washed, and disinfected with an approved EPA disinfectant.
- *Scheduled cleaning* should be done on a regular basis for all wheelchairs and walkers in use, including either manual cleaning and disinfecting or use of automated cleaning and infection control systems.

Oxygen equipment

Oxygen equipment can easily become contaminated and implicated in nosocomial infections. Control includes:

- *Use standard precautions*, including washing hands and wearing gloves when working with oxygen equipment to avoid spreading contamination.
- *Avoid humidification* when possible. Flow rates of 1-4 l/m per mask or nasal cannula allow for adequate humidification from the respiratory tract, but higher flow rates or flow directly to a trachea requires humidification. In-line fine particle nebulizers have become contaminated when oxygen is mixed with ambient air from an oxygen wall outlet.
- *Decondensate* any tubing as needed.
- *Use only sterile solutions* for humidification or inhalation.
- Use *disposable equipment* (regulators, masks, tubing, humidifiers) and replace according to manufacturer's directions. Equipment should never be shared among patients. Nasal cannulas and facemasks should be cleaned regularly as replaced scheduled intervals.
- *Store oxygen cylinders (green tanks) properly* in upright position and only in areas that are designated as clean.

Transfer/discharge planning and Immunizations

Infection control and transfer/discharge planning must be a joint effort so that the transfer and discharge documents provide the information that the individual or staff at transfer facilities need. Information should include:

- Contact telephone numbers/email addresses/street addresses for IPC to contact patient for discharge surveillance and patient or transfer facility staff to contact IPC if problems arise.
- An outline of risk factors for infection incurred during hospital stay, including stay in ICU or specialized units and use of invasive devices, such as central venous lines, ventilators, and/or urinary catheters.
- Information sheets outlining signs of infection for all risk factors, especially if patient is discharged home without nursing care.
- Public Health notification if indicated by local or state regulations.
- Follow-up appointment dates, with physicians or infection control.
- Specific directions for medication or treatments, especially important for antibiotics or wound treatment.

Influenza

Influenza, a viral respiratory disease, is transmitted by person-to-person contact through droplets generated when people sneeze or cough as well as by direct contact with sputum. Those exposed may be infectious the day before symptoms and 5 days after, and outbreaks often affect both staff and patients. The CDC provides guidelines for immunization and treatment of patients exposed to influenza:

- Rapid influenza virus testing done for those with recent onset of symptoms and viral cultures from a subset of patients to identify the virus type and confirm testing results.
- Droplet precautions for all those suspected or confirmed wit influenza, with those suspected separated from those confirmed.
- Current season's vaccination administered to those not immunized.
- Providing influenza antiviral prophylaxis and treatment according to most current recommendations.
- Limiting visitors or posting notices to advise people with symptoms not to visit.

Control of transmission

The patient's immunization status is often neglected and not questioned during the admission procedure, so this information is frequently not in the patient's record. While most people who went to school in the United States were required to have childhood vaccinations, many adults do not take influenza, mumps, measles, chicken pox, hepatitis B or tetanus booster. Many others are not tested for tuberculosis, so immunization of patients is an area of concern for ICPs. The ICP should work with admissions to ensure that all patients are queried about their immunization status, including the last influenza shot and last tetanus booster. When appropriate, patients should be offered immunizations during hospitalization, especially if there is a possibility of exposure to infective agents as occurs with outbreaks. Ideally, immunizations would be given prior to hospitalization, but this involves consistently educating physicians of the need through an ongoing infection control education program.

Biological agents

Organizational plan

The ICP and the infection control team should develop specific plans for dealing with different bioterrorism agents and training should be provided to staff. However, there are similar steps to take regardless of the pathogen. An organized approach should include the following steps:

- Be on the alert for possible bioterrorism-related infections, based on clusters of patients or symptoms.
- Use personal protection equipment, including respirators when indicated.
- Complete thorough assessment of patient, including medical history, physical examination, immunization record, and travel history.
- Provide a probable diagnosis based on symptoms and lab findings, including cultures.
- Provide treatment, including prophylaxis while waiting for laboratory findings.
- Use transmission precautions as well as isolation for suspected biologic agents.
- Notify local, state, and federal authorities as per established protocol.
- Conduct surveillance and epidemiological studies to identify at risk populations.
- Develop plans to accommodate large numbers of patients:
  o Restricting elective admissions.
  o Transferring patients to other facilities.

     o   Reutilizing existing facilities.

Collaboration with public health agencies

Community responses to biologic agents, such as anthrax, smallpox, and influenza, require coordination and planning with public health and other healthcare providers to meet the needs of those infected and to provide information to those who are at risk. Collaborative efforts include planning for:
- Notification of all those involved immediately per telephone/email tree.
- Immunization plans, including availability of vaccines, sites for administration, staffing.
- Education of the public about signs and symptoms and steps to take to prevent becoming infected or spreading infection.
- Training of staff for emergency preparedness/ infection control.
- Stockpiling medications and equipment, such as personal protective equipment, respirators.
- Facilities plan to accommodate large numbers of patients in isolation rooms, including cohorting.
- Environmental monitoring of air and water for contamination.
- Establishing procedures with coroner for handling deaths.
- Epidemiological studies and surveillance.
- Staff assigned to serve as liaison among agencies.

Anthrax

There are a number of different infections that could be part of a bioterrorism attack. The type of barrier/isolation needed is dependent upon the symptoms and the mode of transmission. Knowledge of typical presenting symptoms and prompt precautions are essential to prevent spread of disease. Anthrax (*Bacillus anthracis*) usually occurs from contact with animals, but as a bioterrorism weapon, anthrax would most likely be aerosolized and inhaled. It is not transferred from person to person. There are 3 types:
- Inhalation: fever, cough, fever, shortness of breath, and general debility
- Cutaneous: small non-painful sores that blister and ulcerate with necrosis at the center.
- Gastrointestinal: nausea, vomiting, diarrhea, and abdominal pain.

The inhaled form of anthrax is the most severe with about a 50% mortality rate. The vaccine for anthrax is not yet available to the public.

Precautions:
- Prophylaxis with antibiotics after exposure.
- Standard precautions
- Contact precautions for wounds if there are cutaneous lesions.

Botulism

Clostridium botulinum produces an extremely poisonous toxin that causes botulism. The organism can be aerosolized or used to infect food. There are 3 primary forms of botulisms:
- *Food borne botulism* results from contamination of food. This type poses the greatest threat from bioterrorism. Symptoms usually appear 12-36 hours after ingestion but may be delayed for 2 weeks and include nausea, vomiting, dyspnea, dysphagia, slurred speech, progressive weakness and paralysis

- *Infant botulism* results from *C. botulinum* ingested into the intestinal tract. Constipation, poor feeding, and progressive weakness are presenting symptoms.
- *Wound* botulism results from contamination of open skin, but symptoms are similar to food borne botulism.

Botulism is not transmitted from person to person, but contaminated food has the potential to infect many people, especially if the contaminated food is manufactured and widely distributed.

Precautions:
- Antitoxin after exposure and as early in disease as possible.
- Standard precautions.

Pneumonic plague

Yersinia pestis causes pneumonic plague, which is normally carried by fleas from infected rats but can be aerosolized to use as a biologic weapon. There are 3 forms of plague, but they sometimes occur together and bubonic and septicemic plague can develop into pneumonic, which is the primary concern related to bioterrorism:
- *Bubonic* occurs when a person is bitten by an infected flea.
- *Pneumonic* occurs with inhalation and results in pneumonia with fever, headache, cough, and progressive respiratory failure.
- *Septicemic* occurs when *Y. pestis* invades the bloodstream, often after initial bubonic or pneumonic plague.

Pneumonic plague can spread easily from person to person. There is no vaccine available. Precautions:
- Immediate antibiotics within first 24 hours are necessary, so early diagnosis is critical.
- Prophylaxis with antibiotics may protect those exposed.
- Droplet precautions should be used with appropriate barriers, such as surgical mask.

Smallpox

The variola virus causes smallpox, which has been eradicated worldwide since 1980, but has the potential for use as a biological weapon because people are no longer vaccinated. Smallpox is extremely contagious and has a high mortality rate (about 30%). Flu-like symptoms appear about 7-17 days after exposure with fever, weakness, vomiting and rash that begins on the face and arms and spreads. The rash becomes pustular, crusts, scabs over and then sloughs off, leaving scars. People remain infective from the first rash until all scabs are gone. The disease can spread through contact with infective fluid from lesions or from contact with clothes or bedding. Aerosol spread is theoretically possible. Precautions:
- Vaccination must be done before symptoms appear and as soon as possible after exposure as vaccination after rash appears will not affect the severity of the disease.
- Maximum precautions should be used, which includes the use of gowns and gloves to enter the room and keeping the patient in a patient or cohorted room.

Tularemia

Francisella tularensis causes tularemia, which is usually transmitted from small mammals to humans through insect bites, ingestion of contaminated food or water, inhalation, or handling of infected animals. Although there is no evidence of person-to-person transmission, *F. tularensis* has the potential to be aerosolized for use as in bioterrorism because it is highly infective and requires only about 10 organisms to infect. Flu-like symptoms appear in 3-5 days after exposure and progress to severe respiratory infection and pneumonia. A vaccine for laboratory workers was available until recently, but the FDA is reviewing it at present, so there is no vaccine available now.

- Prophylaxis with antibiotics within 24 hours may prevent disease.
- Standard precautions are sufficient.
- Biologic safety measures should be used for laboratory specimens.
- Autopsy procedures that may cause tissue to be aerosolized should be avoided.

Viral hemorrhagic fevers

Viral hemorrhagic fevers are zoonoses (spread from animals to humans) and comprise a number of different disease: Ebola, Lassa, Marburg, yellow, Argentine and Crimean-Congo. Some hemorrhagic fevers can spread person to person, notably Ebola, Marburg, and Lassa through close contact with body fluids or items contaminated. Hemorrhagic fevers are extremely contagious multi-system diseases, and those in contact with infected patients are at risk of infection   Symptoms vary somewhat according to the disease but present with flu-like symptoms that progress to bleeding under the skin and internally, and some people develop kidney failure and central nervous system symptoms, such as coma and seizures. Treatment is supportive although ribavirin has been used to treat Crimean-Congo hemorrhagic fever. Mortality rates are high. Only yellow fever and Argentine have vaccines. Precautions:

- Maximum precautions must be used with full barrier precautions, with care used in any handling of blood and body fluids or wastes.

Program Management and Communication

Program Planning

Written mission statement, goals, and measurable objectives

The mission statement of the Infection Control Program should identify the program, state its function, and outline the purpose and strategy of the program:

- The mission of the Infection Control Committee of X Hospital, a collaborative group of infection control professionals, physicians, epidemiologists, and support staff, is to promote health and safety of patients, visitors, and staff by decreasing transmission of infections through an organized, comprehensive, and cost-effective surveillance and education program based on outcomes.

The mission statement may be followed by specific tasks of the committee:

- Investigation of outbreaks.
- Development of educational programs.

Goals should be achievable aims, essentially end results, developed for specific units of the facility or the facility in general:

- Reduction in surgical site infections.
- Objectives are the measurable steps taken to achieve goals:
- Audit antibiotic use and establish antibiotic prophylaxis protocol within 6 months.
- Provide monthly staff training in surgical site infection control.

Facility Profile

Patient population

The patient population is an important consideration when developing an infection control plan. There are a number of issues that can impact planning:

- *Size* of the population varies considerably according to the size of the facility. A facility that accommodates 100 patients needs a much different plan than one with 1000 patients.
- *Demographic information* may provide information about risk factors:
  - o Socio-economic status may impact general health, compliance with medical treatments, and follow-up.
  - o ge variations affect risk factors. Neonates pose different problems for infection control than geriatric patients.
  - o Cultural factors, related to ethnicity or country of origin, may pose distinct health problems.
- *Immunocompromised status* poses greater risk of infections. Status may be related to external factors, such as high rates of HIV related to IV drug use, or immunosuppression from drugs related to transplantation, and these types of subgroups represent distinct risk factors.

Major services offered

Major services offered is of primary importance in developing an infection control plan as some types of service carry much higher risks than others.

- *Intensive care units* are consistently cited as high-risk areas because of the severity of the patients' condition as well as the need for invasive devices, such as central venous lines and ventilators.
- *Transplant units* pose special risk because of the immunocompromised status of patients.
- *Surgical service*, by its nature, involves invasive procedures that pose the risk for surgical site and bloodstream infections.
- *Outpatient services* bring a wide variety of patients together and make follow-up difficult.
- *Clinics*, depending upon the type, may bring patients who are very ill or immunocompromised into the facility.
- *High-risk nurseries* have infants with little resistance to infection.
- *Laboratory services* facilitate testing and surveillance if on site but also have risk factors associated with bloodborne pathogens. Off site services may delay testing.

Customer needs and satisfaction

Customer needs and satisfaction can be difficult to define and relate to the infection control plan because they are very individual. Assessment of satisfaction, including opportunities for feedback, must be built into any plan. The assumption may be that the patient is the customer, but with an infection control plan, there are many customers:
- *Hospital administrators* want a plan that is cost-effective and reduces infections and liability.
- *Physicians* want a plan that provides positive outcomes for their patients and assists them in providing care.
- *Nursing staff* want a plan that is practical, efficient, and can be implemented without increasing the work burden.
- *Patients* want to avoid complications and regain their health without worrying about a plan.
- *Environmental services* want a plan that relates to the resources available in the departments.
- *Accreditation agencies* want a plan that provides documented proof of compliance with standards related to infection control.

Number of health care workers

The number of health care workers in a facility has a considerable impact on the planning process for an infection control plan because of the need to train and monitor staff compliance with infection control. One ICP may be able to personally train a staff of 30, but when the staff numbers are in the hundreds with all different levels of expertise, and then there are many issues related to training and monitoring:
- Training sessions are needed at different times of day for people working on different shifts as well as repeat training sessions to accommodate large numbers of staff.
- Different types of training specific to the needs of special areas, such as ICU or HRN, are necessary
- Increased economic resources are needed with large numbers of staff because of costs involved in purchasing or producing training materials and kits.
- IC staff resources needed to provide training along with associated costs increase with numbers of healthcare workers.

Equipment, resources, and personnel

Specific equipment and resources for the infection control program may be overlooked in the budget process but are critically important. Resources include not only personnel in the program but consultants to provide additional information or guidance. A valuable resource for ICPs is membership in state and national organizations, such as the Association for Professionals in Infection Control (APIC) in order to remain keep abreast of current trends and regulations. The ICPs should receive journals, such as *The American Journal of Infection Control* and *The Journal of Hospital Infection.* They must have access to a medical library and reference materials to aid in research and office space and conference rooms for meetings. Basic equipment, such as computers, printers, scanners, and telephones must be available in numbers sufficient for the number of staff. Additional equipment, such as projectors and screens for computer presentations may be needed.

Personnel for the infection control committee vary in number according to the size of the facility and its programs. In 1980, the CDC recommended 1 ICP per every 250 patient beds, but this was before the extensive use of out-patient surgery and shortened hospital stays, which make counting just patients in hospital beds non-representative, so current recommendations are for one ICP for every 100 patient beds. Most committees include physicians who are infection control specialist and/or epidemiologists, but other personnel should include representatives from different major departments in the facility, such as nursing services, laboratory, and environmental services. Additional personnel that may be necessary in large facilities include biostatisticians, research analysts, computer programmers, and office staff. An effective infection control program must have adequate staff to carry out surveillance, analyze results, disseminate results, and train staff. The number and type of personnel must be considered in light of the demands on their time and the tasks to be accomplished.

Hardware and software options

The infection control program must be able to survey, analyze and take action quickly in the event of outbreaks or clusters of infection. Often, infection control is hampered by a lack of integration among existing computer hardware and software programs. The laboratory may use one program: nursing, another. In some facilities, record keeping and reporting is still done by hand. Therefore, the problem of deciding what course to take with hardware and software can be difficult. Ideally, all computer systems and software should be integrated, but this can be very costly. If a facility uses a software designer to create a program specifically meeting the needs of an institution, it may not communicate with reporting or other software. Even if programs and equipment are purchased, they may be subject to expensive updates every couple of years. Some programs are web-based, requiring Internet capability. In many cases, hiring a consultant with expertise in medical hardware and software to advise about the best solution may be the best option.

Meetings of the infection control committee

Facilitating meetings of the infection control committee requires preplanning as well as active guidance during the meeting. Focusing on one or two issues of the action plan may be more productive than trying to discuss all goals and objectives:
- *Send reminders* to committee members, including date and time and a clear outline of what is expected of the member at the meeting, such as giving a report or providing information.
- *Review task lists* from prior meetings to ensure that all issues are covered.
- *Prepare an agenda*, based on the action plan and task lists, to guide the group discussion.
- *Review surveillance data* and prepare reports of any outbreaks or clusters of concern.
- *Copy all pertinent documents/* data reports for committee members.
- *Reserve any necessary equipment,* such as computers or projectors, and arrange for them to be set up and available in the meeting room.
- *Monitor time* and ensure discussions are balanced and each person contributes.

Special projects

<u>Controlling expenditures</u>
Cost-benefit analysis
According to the CDC, a surgical site infection caused by *Staphylococcus aureus* results in an average of 12 additional days of hospitalization and costs $27,000. (In actuality, the cost may vary widely from one institution to another; so local data may be used.) A cost-benefit analysis uses average cost of infection and the cost of intervention to demonstrate savings. For example, if an institution were averaging 10 surgical site infections annually, the cost would be:
$$10 \times \$27,000 = \$270,000 \text{ annually.}$$

If the interventions include new software ($10,000) for surveillance, an additional staff person ($65,000), benefits ($15,000) and increased staff education, including materials ($2000), the total intervention cost would be:
$$\$10,000 + \$65,000 + \$15,000 + \$2000 = \$92,000.00$$

If the goal were to decrease infections by 50% to 5 infections per year, the savings would be calculated:
$$5 \times \$27,000 = \$135,000$$

Subtracting the intervention cost from the savings:
$$\$135,000 - \$92,000 = \$43,000 \text{ annual cost benefit.}$$

Cost-effective analysis, efficacy studies, and product evaluation
Each year, about 2 million nosocomial infections result in 90,000 deaths and an estimated $6.7 billion in additional health costs. From that perspective, decreasing infections should reduce costs, but there are human savings in suffering as well, and it can be difficult to place a dollar value on that. A cost-effective analysis measures the effectiveness of an intervention rather than the monetary savings. If each infection adds about 12 days to hospitalization, then a reduction in infection by 5 would be calculated:
$$5 \times 12 = 60 \text{ fewer patient infection days.}$$

Efficacy studies may compare a series of cost-benefit analyses to determine the intervention with the best cost-benefit. They may also be used for process or product evaluation. For example, a study might be done to determine the infection rates of 4 different types of catheters to determine which type resulted in the fewest infections, thus saving the most money (and infection days). (Incremental cost-effectiveness ratio is the ratio of cost change to outcome change.)

Recommendations based on clinical outcomes and financial implications

Interventions and outcomes should be tied to each other. After an initial cost-benefit analysis and institution of an intervention in infection control, outcomes need to be assessed carefully to determine if the intervention is meeting the goal set for it and is cost-effective. If, for example, the hospital is investing $93,000 additionally each year expecting a savings of 5 infections at $135,000 ($43,000 net), but in fact the savings amount to only 2 infections at $34,000, then the added cost to the hospital is $59,000. Changes in practice, however, cannot be made only on the basis of monetary figures. Further analysis must be done to determine if other variables affected the outcomes. If the hospital opened a transplant unit with additional surgical patients, then the reduction in 2 infections might be impressive. If there is a *staph* carrier among the staff, then this might account for additional infections. In some cases, a change of practice is required.

Cost reduction

Documentation
Many costs associated with infection control are fixed and realistically cannot be recouped; however, infection control is mandated, not optional, so the goal of an infection control program is to use resources as efficiently as possible to lower the infection rate to the point of diminishing returns where there is acceptable reduction of infection rates but further investment is not cost-effective. Documentation requires extensive statistical analysis that includes cost-benefit and cost-effectiveness. Calculations should document monetary savings based on fewer infections and reduction in infection days, theoretically opening the rooms to other patients and increased income, referred to as opportunity costs, which must also be calculated. Any variable costs associated with opportunity costs must be considered. Targeted analysis of specific interventions that show outcomes can help to evaluate the effectiveness of the infection control program. Cost reduction should be demonstrated with graphs, charts, and explanatory text.

Communication and Feedback

Health care workers responsibilities

Health care workers have a primary role in preventing and controlling infections, especially those whose work puts them in direct contact with patients, such as nursing staff in the operating room and nursing units or laboratory technicians. Healthcare workers must be knowledgeable about diseases and disease processes as well as infection control, including signs and symptoms of infections, risk factors, and preventive methods. Specific responsibilities for health care workers include:
- Using proper hand hygiene at all times, including handwashing and use of antiseptic hand cleaner both before and after patient contact.
- Using barrier precautions, including personal protective equipment such as gloves, gowns, and masks or respirators as needed.
- Using aseptic technique and proper procedures for urinary catheters, central venous lines, and other invasive procedures.
- Reporting any indications of infection to the physician and to the infection control committee as per protocol.

Nail care
The subungual (beneath the nails) area of the fingers harbors high levels of microbes, especially *Staphylococcus*, Corynebacteria, Gram-negative rods such as *Pseudomonas* spp. as well as yeast. Both long nails and artificial nails have been implicated in transmission of infections. Because of this, the CDC recommends that healthcare workers who have contact with patients, supplies, medicine, food, or equipment not wear artificial nails or nail tips and keep nails trimmed to about 1/4 inch. Fingernail polish that is freshly applied does not increase bacterial count, but chipped polish can harbor bacteria, so most infection control policies allow either no nail polish or unchipped nail polish. Sequin, rhinestones, or other nail decorations also have the potential to harbor bacteria. While bacteria in the subungual area are most concentrated in the 1 mm closest to the skin, there are other problems associated with long nails:
- Scratching patients.
- Puncturing gloves.
- Interfering with palpation.

Distribution of infection control findings and recommendations

Infection control findings are the result of surveillance activities that may target particular units or in some cases individuals. For this reason, there may be some restriction to access of some or all reports. Part of establishing an infection control program is to determine the reporting tree: who gets which report and how. Typically, all members of the infection control committee would have access to all reports, as would the administration. Reports that related to the entire facility, such as overall infection rates, would be distributed widely. For more sensitive reports, at the next level department chairs would receive reports and recommendations related to their own units and would then disseminate the information as appropriate. Any individual findings, such as surgical site infections for individual surgeons, are usually provided to the department chair and the individual. Dissemination may be in print or by password protected Internet or Intranet postings.

Dissemination of pertinent policies and procedures

Policies, procedures, guidelines, consensus statements, position papers, and standards apply to all staff and should be widely disseminated to all departments. Many institutions now make these types of information available to the public as an ongoing effort to educate the public about infection control and demonstrate the institution's commitment to patient safety. Methods of dissemination include:
- *Print:* Infection control manuals are routinely produced each year and disseminated to all departments and used for staff orientation and training.
- *Internet:* Manuals are now posted on the Internet in facility web pages for easy access. In some cases, the complete manual is posted, but in others, only parts. Some areas of the manual may be password protected to limit access.
- *E-mail:* Both intranet and Internet email can be used to send reports.
- *Intranet:* Facilities that have an internal Intranet routinely post the infection control manual on the intranet so that it can be easily accessed within the facility to be used for reference and training.

Communicating resource needs to administration

In an era of increasing medical costs and decreasing reimbursement, communicating infection control resource needs to administration requires careful planning and statistical analysis to support the need and the cost-effectiveness of the resources, outlining exactly how the resources are going to improve infection control. Strategies include:
- *Statistical support*, including cost-benefit and cost-effectiveness analysis to demonstrate value of the resource in controlling infection. The use of charts and diagrams is effective as a tool to present information clearly.
- *Research support* can include a literature review and summary of reports and research supporting the use of the resource.
- *Demonstrations* that allow the administration to see the resource and view its use can be persuasive.
- *Staff support* from other healthcare workers, such as physicians or nurses, who recognize the need may bolster an argument in favor of a resource.

Consultation

Infection control is central to patient safety and any changes in a facility, whether it is a change of product or procedure or a renovation project, has the potential to increase transmission of disease; therefore, an ICP should be a standing member available for consultation of any committee or group

- 122 -

whose actions may impact patient care. The ICP should be knowledgeable about the issues and be prepared to research and provide guidance. Risk management professionals protect the institution from liability related to patient injury, including infections, and it is critical that risk management have as clear an understanding of causes related to an infection as possible. The ICP may use tracer methodology to identify possible sources of transmission and to determine if processes were used correctly in an effort to prevent infection because this information can help to support or deny liability, allowing risk management to make decisions about a case.

Annual summaries

The annual summary is an important tool for the ICP because it clearly outlines the progress (or lack) in infection control over the year. Since outcomes are of primary importance, the summary should utilize the infection control plan and be organized in the same way, listing the goal, the objectives (actions), and the specific outcomes related to those objectives. Each goal and objective should be included, even if no action took place. Statistical analysis should be completed prior to beginning the annual summary, and the analyses should be included in the document. Charts, graphs, and diagrams, such as line and bar graphs, flow charts, decision trees, and cause and effect diagrams should be part of the summary. The summary should highlight achievements and list ongoing or potential goals for the following year. A separate timeline that gives a brief summary of action month by month may also be included.

Liaison officer duties

The role of liaison officer is an integral part of the ICP's responsibilities, especially with the increase of outpatient surgery and short hospital stays, sending patients home or into extended care facilities. Communication among the different agencies and facilities caring for patients is necessary if infection control surveillance and preventive methods are to be accurate and effective. It's especially important that the ICP serve as liaison to feeder institutions, such as small hospitals that transfer patients into a larger facility and extended care facilities to which discharge patients are transferred. Having an assigned ICP to serve as liaison and to meet regularly with other agencies/ facilities allows the ICP to serve as a consultant so that shared goals and objectives can be developed. Maintaining a close working relationship with the public health department is necessary because of reporting requirements and the need for cooperation in the event of outbreaks or pandemics.

Marketing and promoting the infection control plan

Providing an infection control plan is only the beginning of marketing and promoting, which must be ongoing endeavors. Some marketing strategies include:
- Patient information sheets telling patients about infection controls standards and procedures and what they should expect from the staff, such as handwashing before and after every contact.
- Maintaining a high profile by visiting different departments and units, talking to staff, asking and answering questions.
- Monthly or weekly promotions, such as slogans, posters and flyers about hand washing throughout the facility.
- Joint activities and promotions with other agencies/facilities in the area.
- Mini-conferences with speakers about infection control issues and vendor displays.
- Regularly-scheduled training sessions for staff and other healthcare workers in the area.
- Events with participative activities, such as handwashing contests with glow-in-the-dark powders or solutions to determine effectiveness of handwashing technique.
- Infection control crossword puzzles or games.
- Newsletters to staff and community about infection control issues.

Advising administration

Initial planning
Construction and renovation pose serious risks to both patients and staff because of the danger of dust and water contamination; therefore, the administration must be advised of all the implications when these projects are undertaken as there are often considerable expenses beyond construction costs in preventing transmission of disease. The American Institute of Architects (AIA) Academy of Architecture for Health publishes guidelines that are used by the CDC and states as minimum standards for construction and renovation in a health care facility. These guidelines require input from the ICP at all stages of construction, including planning that includes an infection control risk assessment (ICRA). The ICP helps to identify support structures that will be needed during construction. Based on the ICRA, a comprehensive plan for renovation and construction should be developed that includes all of the necessary elements to carry out the project while ensuring infection control monitoring and patient safety.

Planning issues
The ICP and administration must deal with a number of issues related to construction:
- Preventing environmental contamination:
    - Construction areas must be sealed off with heavy plastic or drywall.
    - Negative pressure must be maintained in construction area.
    - Outdoor windows and doors may need to be sealed..
    - Additional filters/ventilation may be required.
    - Foot traffic should be directed around construction.
    - Cleaning of construction site and removing debris must be done daily.
- Protecting patients:
    - Patient units may be closed.
    - Patients, especially those at high risk, may be transferred away from construction areas.
    - Patient transportation should be limited.
    - Additional surveillance may be required.
- Incorporating infection control into construction design.
    - Walls, floors, and surfaces should be easy to clean and resistant to disinfectant and water damage.
    - Adequate handwashing facilities and space for sharps disposal must be available.
    - Positive and/or negative pressure airflow should be planned as needed by the type of construction project.

Advice to contractors

The ICP must work very closely with contractors to assure that they understand infection control implications of construction and that they follow guidelines, including the construction of adequate plastic or drywall barriers. Often the ICP and contractor will work together with a consultant who is an expert in medical construction, and the ICP must ensure that recommendations are followed. The ICP must regularly monitor the construction site for compliance or problems. Agreements about construction cleanup both during and after construction should be made. The CDC advises that mandatory adherence agreements for infection control be part of construction contracts. Contractors must understand what the penalties are for noncompliance and what steps they must take to correct problems. Additionally, the ICP and contractor should review plans for construction worker safety and OSHA guidelines, ensuring that workers are protected from potential danger and infection during demolition or construction.

Job description

Job descriptions are often vague documents that list generalities but do not adequately represent the actual requirements of a position, but in order to get properly qualified staff, a job description should be up-to-date and accurate and include the following:

- *General job description* that states the major areas of responsibility. Some infection control positions include other responsibilities, such as employee health or inservice training, and this should be clear. The work schedule (times and days) should be outlined.
- *Qualifications,* including the type of degree(s), licenses and/or certification that is required. Desired work experience should be included, such as 3 years of experience in infection control. This may also include a section about the ability to demonstrate knowledge, such as "demonstrates knowledge of epidemiology."
- *Salary and benefits,* such as insurance and vacation time.
- *Duties* that are expected. This should be a comprehensive list that lists specific activities, such as conducting surveillance, providing staff training, and preparing the annual report.

Goals for professional development

Identifying goals for professional development and ongoing education of infection control personnel requires a commitment on the part infection control to remain current and on the part of the facility administration to provide financial support or incentives, such as advancement in pay for those who continue their education, tuition assistance, and release time. The goals of both professional development and ongoing education are for staff to be knowledgeable and informed with expertise in the area of infection control and epidemiology. Professional development can include membership in national organizations, attending regional or national conferences, or taking courses in traditional classes or through the Internet. One goal of any infection control program should be for staff to complete certification for infection control professionals. If not already required as a qualification for the job of infection control professional, completing this certification within a year or two may be a condition of hiring.

Consultation to management

The ICP consults with management regarding the Exposure Control Plan for occupational infections/exposures. OSHA defines occupational exposure as "reasonably anticipated skin, eye, mucous membrane, or parenteral contact with blood or other potentially infectious materials" resulting from performance of duties. Further, any employer with employee(s) with such occupational exposure must have a written Exposure Control Plan, which aims to minimize or eliminate danger to the employee(s). This plan must include:

- Documented input from staff involved in direct patient care.
- schedule and methods of compliance, such as Hepatitis B vaccination programs
- Methods of communicating hazards to staff.
- Record keeping.
- Procedures for investigating exposure incidents that might result in infection.
- nnual review and update to reflect technology changes or safer medical devices.
- n exposure determination that includes listing of all job classifications with exposures and the types of exposures.

- Methods of compliance with OSHA standards, including hand hygiene, barrier precautions, sharps disposal methods.

Compliance with regulations and standards

There is a maze of regulations and standards that must be reconciled and complied with, and this task falls within the responsibilities of the ICP. Various regulating agencies include:
- *State and local government* regulations may overlap other agencies because most states rely on other regulatory agencies, such as the FDA and CDC for medical standards although standards related to kitchens, food preparation, and sanitation may vary somewhat.
- *Hospital Infection Control Practices Advisory Committee (HICPAC)* works with the CDC to establish standards and guideline.
- *CDC* is central to prevention of control of infections and issues standards and procedures for preventing transmission, such as barrier precautions, isolation guidelines, and TB monitoring, and disease reporting.
- *OSHA* regulates occupational health issues related to exposure to infectious materials.
- *FDA* regulates medications and medical devices, including recall and reuse issues.
- *Joint Commission* accredits hospitals and medical facilities and requires extensive documented compliance with standards.

Obtaining and maintaining accreditation/licensure

Obtaining accreditation and licensure is based on meeting standards set by a regulatory agency. The Joint Commission evaluates many aspects of the facility, including infection control, for accreditation. The guidelines by which hospitals are evaluated are often very specific, such as the exact time in minutes or hours after admission for pneumonia that a patient receives an antibiotic, with scores according to the elapsed time. The infection control professional must review, understand, communicate, and establish guidelines for all accreditation requirements to ensure that the various staff and departments are aware of the requirements and are documenting compliance. Because the accreditation survey utilizes tracer methodology, which evaluates the processes that are in place, extensive staff training regarding processes at all levels must be completed. Additionally, the ICP can use tracer methodology as part of infection control, allowing staff to understand and practice the type of information they need to supply to the accreditation team.

Influencing policymaking bodies

The ICP is in a unique position to influence policymaking within an institution, but even more important is the ability to influence policymaking at a state or national level. The ICP should take an active role in national organizations that promote the development of consistent standards and participation in the political process. Three organizations have cooperated to create model legislation that can serve as a template for state legislatures adopting regulations regarding collecting and reporting of data regarding hospital-acquired infection:
- *The Association for Professionals in Infection Control and Epidemiology (APIC)* (11,000 members), open to physicians, epidemiologists, nurses, laboratory technicians, and others involved in reducing the risk of infection.
- *The Infectious Disease Society of America (IDSA)* (8000 members), open to scientists, physicians, and others specialize in infectious diseases.

- *The Society for Healthcare Epidemiology of America (SHEA)* (1200 members), open to those with a doctorate or master's degree in a healthcare field, 5 years experience, or SHEA certification and promotes healthcare epidemiology.

Communicating changes in regulations and standards

Communication of changes in regulations and standards must be made in a timely manner and disseminated widely, especially in the changes result in differences in processes or procedures. The ICP is often the first person to receive information about pending changes and should begin early to make plans to communicate to others. There are a number of ways to communicate changes:
- *Infection Control Plan* should be updated on an annual basis to include all information related to changes in regulations and standards.
- *Consulting with administration* about impending changes and courses of action.
- *Staff meetings* with department heads and staff who are directly impacted by changes to outline changes.
- *Print materials*, such as documents, fliers, and posters should be prepared to provide the necessary information.
- *Email* communications can quickly alert staff to changes.
- *Training classes* that cover new standards should be provided as quickly as possible.

Reporting communicable diseases

Mechanisms for reporting of communicable diseases vary somewhat from state to state, but there are city, county, state, national, and international reporting regulations. The ICP will normally notify the local and state authorities of communicable diseases, and the state, in turn, notifies the CDC, which may notify WHO for internationally reportable diseases, such as smallpox or polio. The CDC maintains a reportable disease list, which is upgraded and revised as necessary and reissued July 1 of each year. It includes infections of concern, such as HIV and HBV. Each state also maintains a reportable disease list, which may or may not be identical with that of the CDC, so the ICP must be familiar with all reportable disease requirements. Much data at the state and local level is confidential name-based information, but data collected at the CDC is without names or personal identifying information. Some states require reporting of hospital-acquired infections.

Assessing infection control implications of pending legislation

When hospital-acquired infections first became reportable, confidentially was a cornerstone, protecting the reporting institution from liability; however, in response to morbidity, mortality, and costs associated with hospital-acquired infections, increasingly states are passing new laws requiring public reporting. Because there is no national standard, the laws, including definitions and types of reporting, vary considerably. In response, APIC, SHEA, and IDSA have proposed legislation to try to standardize reporting requirements. As reports become public, in some cases with hospital-specific data, there is tremendous pressure on the ICP to reduce rates of infection. At present, 6 states (Florida, Illinois, Missouri, New York, Pennsylvania, Virginia) require public reporting of data. Nebraska and Nevada require reporting that is not available to the public. Bills regarding reporting are under study or being considered in about 20 other states, with more expected to follow suit. The ICP must be familiar with current or pending legislation and keep the administration appraised, taking early steps toward compliance.

Quality-Performance Improvement

Continuous Quality Improvement

Continuous Quality Improvement (CQI) emphasizes the organization and systems and processes within that organization rather than individuals. It recognizes internal customers (staff) and external customers (patients) and utilizes data to improve processes. CQI represents the concept that most processes can be improved. CQI uses the scientific method of experimentation to meet needs and improve services and utilizes various tools, such as brainstorming, multivoting, various charts and diagrams, storyboarding, and meetings. Core concepts include:
- Quality and success is meeting or exceeding internal and external customer's needs and expectations.
- Problems relate to processes, and variations in process lead to variations in results.
- Change can be in small steps.

Steps to CQI include:
- Forming a knowledgeable team.
- Identifying and defining measures used to determine success.
- Brainstorming strategies for change.
- Plan, collect, and utilize data as part of making decisions.
- Test changes and revise or refine as needed.

Shewhart cycle (Plan-Do-Check-Act)

The Shewhart cycle (Plan-Do-Check-Act) is a method of continuous improvement that is part of quality management and is used to solve problems:
- *Plan* involves identifying and analyzing the problem clearly defining the problem, setting goals, and establishing a process that coordinates with coordinates with leadership. Extensive brainstorming, including fishbone diagrams, identifies problematic processes and lists current process steps. Data is collected and analyzed and root cause analysis completed.
- *Do* involves generating solutions from which to select one or more and then implementing the solution on a trial basis.
- *Check* involves gathering and analyzing data to determine the effectiveness of the solution. If effective, then continue to *Act*; if not, return to *Plan* and pick a different solution.
- *ct* involves identifying changes that need to be done to fully implement solution, adopting solution and continuing to monitor results while picking another improvement project.

Graphic tools

Ishikawa "fishbone" diagram
The Ishikawa "fishbone" diagram resembling the head and bones of a fish, is an analysis tool to determine causes and effects. In infection control, it is used to help identify root causes. Typically, the "head" is labeled with the problem (the effect). Then, each bone is labeled with a category (causes), traditionally M (used for manufacturing), P (used for administration and service), and S (used for service).
- M: methods, materials, manpower, machines, measurement, mother nature (environment).
- P: people, prices, promotion, places, policies, procedures, product.
- S: surroundings, suppliers, systems, skills.

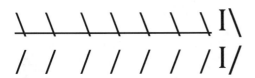

The categories serve only as a guide and can be selected and modified as needed. For example, if the effect is urinary tract infections, then all possible causes, derived from brainstorming, would be listed on the "bones": people, places, product, surroundings, material Then, each category listed would be questioned: "What are the issues affecting this category?" "What is the problem?" "Why is it happening?"

Pareto chart
A Pareto chart is a combination vertical bar graph and line graph. Typically, bar graph values are arranged in descending order. For example, if incidences of bloodstream infections were being plotted by unit, the unit with the largest number would be first on the left. A line graph superimposed over the bar graph usually shows what accumulated percentage of the total is represented by the elements of the bar graph. Thus, if 50 infections occurred in ICU and that represented 30% of the total, the line graph would start at 30%. If 40 infections occurred in the transplant unit (24% of total), the line graph would show 54% at the bar for the transplant unit. The Pareto chart helps to demonstrate the most common causes or sources of problems and has given rise to the 80/20 rule: 80% of the problem often derives from 20% of causes.

Flow chart
A flow chart is a tool of quality improvement and is used to provide a pictorial/ schematic representation of a process. It is a particularly helpful tool for quality improvement projects when each step in a process is analyzed when searching for solutions to a problem. Typically, the following symbols are used:
- Parallelogram: Input and output (start/end)
- rrow: Direction of flow
- Diamond-shape: Conditional decision (Yes/No or True/False)
- Circles: connectors with diverging paths with multiple arrows coming in but only one going out.

A variety of other symbols may be used as well to indicate different functions. Flow goes from top to bottom and left to right. Flow charts are particularly helpful to help people to visualize how a process is carried out and to examine a process for problems. Flow charts may also be used to plan a process before it's utilized.

Identifying opportunities for improvement

Opportunities for improvement may be evident on analysis of indicators (typical causes of infection, such as central venous lines) and outcomes (rates of infection). Through surveillance activities, both numerator and denominator data is produced and these outcomes should be measured against internal benchmarks that have been established, or external benchmarks, such as national rates of infection. Once it is clear where variances lie, then these particular indicators can be targeted for improvement. Additionally, other findings or observations may indicate the need for changes in processes. For example, cost-benefit analysis may show that some procedures or processes are not cost-effective and there may be a number of different solutions that might achieve the same or better results. These procedures or process may be reviewed and alternate solutions sought so that these processes or procedures become a target for reduction in variable costs to a facility.

Multidisciplinary quality/performance strategies

Continuous Quality Improvement (CQI) is a multidisciplinary management philosophy that can be applied to all aspects of business, whether related to infection control, purchasing, or human resources issues. The skills used for epidemiologic research (data collection, analysis, outcomes, action plans) are all applicable to analysis of non-infectious events because they are based on solid scientific methods. Multi-disciplinary planning can bring valuable insights from various perspectives, and strategies used in one context can often be applied to another. Increasingly, infection control must be concerned with cost-effectiveness as the costs of medical care continue to rise, so the ICP is not in an isolated position in an institution but is just one part of the whole, facing similar concerns as those in other disciplines. Disciplines are often interrelated in their functions. For example, Human Resources hires personnel, but the ICP monitors and trains them for compliance with infection control standards. Purchasing may order catheters, but the type may affect infection rates.

Patient safety performance improvement activities

Patient safety performance improvement activities are those that are designed as campaigns to reduce error or improve patient outcomes, such as reduction in infection. Often the activities are targeted to one group (such as physicians) or one type of patient, but they may also be broader. Because performance improvement and processes are central to the Joint Commission's accreditation standards, those standards make a good beginning point to look at possible improvement activities as well as the data that has been collected. Many problems are multidisciplinary and may involve, for example, both environmental services and infection control, such as the need to increase hepatitis B vaccinations in housekeeping staff. Teams must decide what to measure, collect data, determine solutions, and then implement solutions in a concerted effort. Patient safety performance activities may include such activities as monitoring air flow to negative-pressure rooms or placing hand antiseptics in every room.

Education

Education

Assessing the educational needs of health care workers

There are a number of different methods that the ICP can use to assess the educational needs of health care workers pertaining to infection control:

- Review job descriptions to determine the educational qualifications/ certifications for all different levels of staff to determine what, realistically, they should be expected to know about infection control.
- Review job orientation and training materials to determine what staff have been taught about infection control.
- Conduct meetings with staff in different departments to brainstorm areas of concern and potential training needs.
- Meet with team leaders and department heads for their input about the need for infection control education.
- dminister short infection control quizzes to staff asking about standard infection control methods, such as barrier precautions and hand washing to determine basic knowledge.
- Provide questionnaires to staff to obtain information about their own perceptions of what they know or need to know about infection control.
- Make direct observations of staff.

Goals, measurable objectives, and lesson plans

Once a topic for infection control education has been chosen, then goals, measurable objectives with strategies, and lesson plans must be developed. A class should stay focused on one area rather than trying to cover many things. For example:

- Goal: increase compliance with hand hygiene standards in ICU.
- Objectives:
  - Develop series of posters and fliers by June 1.
  - Observe 100% compliance with hand hygiene standards at 2 weeks, 1 month, and 2 month intervals after training is completed.
- Strategies:
  - Conduct 4 classes at different times over a one-week period, May 25-31.
  - Place posters in all nursing units, staff rooms, and utility rooms by January 3.
  - Develop PowerPoint presentation for class and Intranet/Internet for access by all staff by May 25.
  - Utilize handwashing kits.
- Lesson plans:
  - Discussion period: Why do we need 100% compliance?
  - PowerPoint: The case for hand hygiene.
  - Discussion: What did you learn?
  - Demonstration and activities to show effectiveness
  - Handwashing technique.

Teaching approaches

Principles of adult learning

Adults come to work with a wealth of life and employment experiences. Their attitudes toward education may vary considerably. There are, however, some principles of adult learning and typical characteristics of adult learners that an instructor should consider when planning strategies for teaching:

- *Practical and goal-oriented:*
    - Provide overviews or summaries and examples.
    - Use collaborative discussions with problem-solving exercises.
    - Remain organized with the goal in mind.
- *Self-directed:*
    - Provide active involvement, asking for input.
    - Allow different options toward achieving the goal.
    - Give them responsibilities.
- *Knowledgeable:*
    - Show respect for their life experiences/ education.
    - Validate their knowledge and ask for feedback.New material to information with which they are familiar.
    - *Relevancy-oriented:*How information will be applied on the job.
    - Clearly identify objectives.
- *Motivated:*
    - Provide certificates of professional advancement and/or continuing education credit when possible.

Audience size and available resources

There are a number of issues related to audience size that must be considered when planning presentations.

- Class participation is more difficult in a large class because there may not be time for all to speak individually. Breaking the class into small groups or pairs for discussion for part of the class time can increase participation, but there must be a focused purpose to the discussion so that people stay on task.
- In small groups, placing chairs in a circle or sitting around a table allows people to look at each other and have more active discussions than if they are sitting in rows.
- Online "virtual" classes can vary considerably in size, depending upon the type of presentation and whether or not scores and replies are automated or posted by the instructor. If a large group is taking an online course, setting up a "chat room" can facilitate exchange of ideas.

Handouts

Handouts are a fixture in classes, but many end up in the wastebasket without ever being used, so thought should be given to providing handouts that are useful:

- Handouts that simply copy a PowerPoint presentation or repeat everything in the presentation are less helpful than those that summarize the main points.
- Giving out handouts immediately prior to a discussion ensures that most of the class will be looking at the handout instead of the speaker. Thus, handouts should be placed in a folder or binder and passed out before class so people can peruse them in advance or passed out at the end of class.
- Handouts can be used to provide guidance or worksheets for small group discussions.
- Poster-type handouts (with drawings or pictures) that can be placed on bulletin boards are useful.

- Handouts should be easily readable and not smudged copies of newspaper articles or small print text.

Audiovisuals

There are a number of issues that must be considered when teaching a course and determining the appropriate audiovisuals and handout materials.

The physical environment is a major consideration, especially when using audiovisual material.

- First, everyone in the room must be able to hear and see. In a small room, a television screen may suffice, but in a large space, a projection screen must be used.
- Another issue is lighting. Some projectors have low resolution and the lights need to be turned off /dimmed or windows covered. Turning lights on and off a dozen times during a presentation can be very distracting. A small portable light at a speaker podium or and alternate presentation can be used.
- Text size for presentations is another issue: PowerPoint or other presentations that include text must be of sufficient font size to be read from the back of the room.

It is impractical to believe that the ICP can produce all educational materials, but careful consideration must be given to a number of issues:

- *Price* ranges from free to hundreds or even thousands of dollars for educational materials, which may be handouts, videos, posters, or entire courses or series of courses available online. The ICP must first consider the budget and then look for material within those monetary constraints. Government agencies, such as the CDC, often have posters and handouts as well as PowerPoint presentations and videos available for download online at no cost.
- *Quality* varies considerably as well. The ICP should consider the goal and objectives before choosing materials, and the materials should be evaluated to determine if they cover all needed information in a clear and engaging manner.
- *Currency* must be considered as well. If material will soon be outdated because of changes in regulations, then it will have to be replaced.

Educational workshops

There are many approaches to teaching, and the ICP must prepare, present, and coordinate a wide range of educational workshops, lectures, discussions, and one-on-one instructions on a variety of infection control topics. Planning time for classes should be made as part of the infection control plan, but allowing for flexibility to contend with unexpected needs. All types of classes will be needed, depending upon the purpose and material:

- *Educational workshops* are usually conducted with small groups, allowing for maximal participation and are especially good for demonstrations and practice sessions.
- *Lectures* are often used for more academic or detailed information that may include questions and answers but limits discussion. An effective lecture should include some audiovisual support.
- *Discussions* are best with small groups so that people can actively participate. This is a good for problem-solving.
- *One-on-one instruction* is especially helpful for targeted instruction in procedures for individuals.
- *Computer/Internet modules* are good for independent learners.

Instructing and advising staff on policy changes

Changes in policies, procedures, or working standards are common and, the ICP is responsible for educating the staff about changes related to infection control, which should be communicated to staff in an effective and timely manner:

- *Policies* are usually changed after a period of discussion and review by administration and staff, so all staff should be made aware of policies under discussion. Preliminary information should be disseminated to staff regarding the issue during meetings or through printed notices.
- *Procedures* may be changed to increase efficiency or improve patient safety often as the result of surveillance and data about outcomes. Procedures changes are best communicated in workshops with demonstrations. Posters and handouts should be available as well.
- *Working standards* are often changed because of regulatory or accrediting requirements and this information should be covered extensively in a variety of different ways: discussions, workshops, handouts so that the implications are clearly understood.

Learner outcomes

When the ICP plans an educational offering, whether it be a class, an online module, a workshop, or educational materials, the ICP should identify learner outcomes, which should be conveyed to the learners from the very beginning so that they are aware of the expectations. The subject matter of the educational material and the learner outcomes should be directly related. For example, if the ICP is giving a class on decontamination of the environment, then a learner outcome might be: "Identify the difference between disinfectants and antiseptics." There may be one or multiple learner outcomes, but part of the assessment at the end of the learning experience should be to determine if, in fact, the learner outcomes have been achieved. A survey of whether or not the learners felt that they had achieved the learner outcomes can give valuable feedback and guidance to the ICP.

Behavior modification and compliance rate
Education, like all interventions, must be evaluated for effectiveness. Two determinants of effectiveness are measures of behavior modification and compliance rates. Behavior modification involves thorough observation and measurement, identifying behavior that needs to be changed and then planning and instituting interventions to modify that behavior. Procedures an ICP can use include demonstrations of appropriate behavior, reinforcement, and monitoring until new behavior is adopted consistently. This is especially important when longstanding procedures, and habits of behavior, are changed. Compliance rates are often determined by observation, which should be done at intervals and on multiple occasions. Outcomes is another measure of compliance; that is, if education is intended to improve patient safety and decrease infection rates and that occurs, it is a good indication that there is compliance. Compliance rates are calculated by determining the number of events/procedures and degree of compliance. This may be determined through observation or record review.

Orientation program for health care workers

The ICP's participation in the facility's orientation program for health care workers is extremely important because it signals the administrative commitment to infection control. Because of that, the ICP presentations should not be relegated to just stand alone "Infection Control" orientation classes but should be integrated with other presentations so that the new hires understand how infection control is a multidisciplinary focus of the institution. Certainly, hand hygiene and use of barrier precautions must be covered in detail as well as information about surveillance and indicators. They must understand the processes in place for both patient and staff safety, but health care workers also need to know what action Human Resources will take if new staff are out of compliance with infection control measures. They should also know, for example what housekeeping does to control infection and what precautions maintenance and food workers use.

Disseminating information on infection control

Dissemination of pertinent information and literature on infection control should be an ongoing scheduled process, at least monthly. The easiest way to disseminate this type of information is through newsletters, either print or electronic.

- *Print newsletters* involve costs that must be considered as part of operating expenses. There is also staff time involved in preparing the document as well as copyright considerations. Most government publications are copyright exempt and can be reproduced, but articles of interest from journals require permission, which may be difficult to obtain for new material. An alternative method is for someone to write a review of an article or articles, including a summary of the main points. Use of pictures adds expense, especially if they are in color.
- *Electronic newsletters* involve staff time but are considerably less expensive. Additionally, links to online articles and color pictures can be easily inserted into the newsletter.

Assessing educational needs of patients/families

There are a number of ways to assess educational needs of patients/families regarding infection control. Using multiple strategies provides the most accurate results:

- *Consult with the public health department* about community issues of infection, such as rates of HBV, HIV, and TB, to determine shared educational needs.
- *Conduct mail surveys* either of the general populace or targeted surveys of former patients and families. Mail survey return rates are often low, so a large number of surveys must be prepared.
- *Conduct telephone surveys* of the same groups, usually with better response and lower costs, but they are time-consuming and may require hiring temporary staff.
- *Conduct onsite surveys* for both inpatients and clinic patients, including both patients and family members. When surveys are requested by staff directly, return rates are good.
- *Conduct Interviews* for inpatients, clinic patients, and families, giving the chance for people to elaborate but requiring much staff time.

Instructing patients/families

Methods to instruct patients and families to prevent and control infections depend on many variables, which may include:

- *Goal:* instruction should be provided keeping the purpose in mind, whether it is to increase handwashing or promote vaccinations.
- *Necessity:* If the patient has a wound or invasive device that requires home care, then intensive one-on-one demonstration and observation is required, but if the need is more general, then fliers or handouts might be sufficient.
- *Educational background:* If most of the hospital population is from an affluent well-educated group, then detailed print information may be indicated. If there is a large illiterate or poorly educated population, then posters or handouts with pictures and little text might be more appropriate.
- *Language:* If there are sufficient populations of non-English speakers, then instructive materials may need to be produced in Spanish, Russian, Chinese, or other languages, or with primarily pictures/drawings.

Public educator role

The ICP is in a unique position to serve as a consultant and educator for the community regarding infectious illness. There are many avenues that the ICP can explore:

- *Schools and universities* present a many opportunities from demonstrating handwashing to small children in elementary school to speaking with students in medical fields to giving lectures on infectious diseases in university classes or public seminars.
- *Service organizations* often invite speakers to discuss topics of interest, and this presents an opportunity to discuss infectious disease issues and to enlist the aid of other organizations in spreading information.
- *News media* is especially interested in information during times of outbreaks, but they may also be willing to interview or allow reports on a regular basis.
- *Job fairs* present an opportunity to speak to a wide range of people about the field of infection control.
- *Unions* may be interested in field-related information about infection control.

Research

Conducting literature search

While there is still a place for research in a medical library that has the latest journals and materials, the reality is that almost all current information can be obtained with an online search; however, access to some journals may require membership in organizations or online subscriptions, and these should be included in the infection control budget for resources because research is critical if the ICP is to stay current and anticipate trends. Information sources include:
- *Journals* sponsored by national or other organizations:
  - *Clinical Infectious Diseases* (IDSA)
  - *The Journal of Infectious Diseases* (IDSA)
  - *merican Journal of Infection Control* (APIC)
  - *Infection Control and Hospital Epidemiology* (SHEA)
  - *Journal of the American Medical Association* (AMA)
  - *New England Journal of Medicine* (Massachusetts Medical Society)
- *Government website* with information of interest.
  - State websites for Departments of Health.
  - CDC: http://www.cdc.gov/ncidod/dhqp/index.html
  - FDA: http://www.fda.gov/
  - OSHA: http://www.osha.gov/
  - NiOSH: http://www.cdc.gov/niosh/

Evaluating research

There are a number of steps to critical reading to evaluate research:
- *Consider the source* of the material. If it is in the popular press, it may have little validity compared to something published in a juried journal.
- *Review the author's credentials* to determine if a person is an expert in the field of study.
- *Determine thesis*, or the central claim of the research. It should be clearly stated.
- *Examine the organization* of the article, whether it is based on a particular theory, and the type of methodology used.
- *Review the evidence* to determine how it is used to support the main points. Look for statistical evidence and sample size to determine if the findings have wide applicability.
- *Evaluate* the overall article to determine if the information seems credible and useful and should be communicated to administration and/or staff.

Incorporation of research findings into practice

Incorporating research findings should be central to all work of the ICP and should be routinely disseminated as part of practice, education and consultation. Any time the ICP gives a presentation or provides written material, references should be made to research findings because this provides supporting evidence and lends credence to the information the ICP is providing. Often research can provide guidance for surveillance or interventions and give valuable insights. References that are used or referred to should always be properly cited so that the work of researchers is credited. If a presentation is given orally, then the ICP should prepare a list of references. Newsletters and e-mail or Internet reports and communications should include research highlights or summaries of current studies of interest, with links to online articles provided when possible to encourage people to read the research for themselves and become more knowledgeable about issues of infection control.

Infection Control Aspects of Employee Health

Pre-placement screening and immunizations

There are a number of issues regarding pre-employment screening, such as screening for criminal records and drug use, but among those concerns, screening for immune status is extremely important for all those employed within a healthcare facility because one healthcare worker can infect many patients, and lack of immunity places the healthcare worker at risk as well. Issues to consider include:

- *Proof of immune status:* Will verbal history be sufficient or must medical records be provided to prove immunization? Which diseases must be included? What testing for immune status will be provided?
- *Immunizations:* Will immunizations be required or voluntary? Which immunizations? What forms are necessary?
- *Service area:* How will immunization requirements vary from one service area to another? Will all staff be required to have some immunizations?
- *Special circumstances:* How will screening and immunizations be done for people who are immunocompromised, HIV positive, or pregnant?

Recommended policies and procedures for pre-placement screening of health care workers are based on guidelines of the American Hospital Association, the Joint Commission, OSHA, and the CDC:

- ckground check and drug testing (required by Joint Commission).
- Worker provides dates of 2 doses of measles, mumps and rubella vaccinations (MMR) and verbal report of varicella or submits for serology testing.
- Workers in contact with blood, body fluids, or body tissue must provide evidence of positive antibodies to HBV or be offered HBV vaccinations. HBV vaccinations cannot be required but non-immunized staff can be prevented from working in high-risk areas.
- Two-step TB skin testing (recommended by OSHA) 1-3 weeks apart. Chest x-ray is required for positive skin testing.
- Immunizations required for all healthcare facility workers should include: MMR, varicella, HBV, and influenza. Tetanus toxoid should be current.

Screening programs

While employment pre-screening requirements focuses on new workers, often other healthcare workers were hired before immunization requirements or are in need of retesting and re-immunization, so the ICP needs to develop programs for screening. Depending upon the number of workers involved, there are different approaches that can be used:

- *Anniversary date* reviews for all staff can include a health update and screening for infectious diseases and immunizations as needed.
- *Department and/or unit* review of all staff in that area can be done during a prescribed period of time with the department chair or supervisor ensuring that all staff are notified and screened.
- *Screening and immunization drives* can be done for 1-2 weeks periods once or twice a year with notices to all employees to participate.
- *Flu shot drives* can be done yearly prior to flu season. Placing staff and tables near staff lounges or dining areas to provide immunizations reminds staff and saves staff time.

Investigation and follow-up

Healthcare worker (HCW) exposure to communicable diseases can be from droplets, airborne particles, or contact with blood or body fluids. There are a number of issues involved in investigation and follow-up after exposure. The most common exposure is through injury with contaminated sharps, such as needles, putting people at risk for HIV, HBV, and HCV especially. The type of exposure and the disease determine the steps to be taken.

- Immediate reporting of all potential exposure, such as needlestick injuries or infectious diagnoses, must be done so that steps can be taken to determine the degree of exposure and steps to prevent infection.
- Contact investigations may need to be completed, especially for airborne or droplet exposure, to ensure that all those in contact with the infected person are notified.
- HCW may need to be removed from duty or patient contact during incubation period.
- Prophylaxis, immunizations, or treatment may be initiated.
- Periodic re-testing may be necessary.

Exposure to communicable diseases

Exposure to HIV

The CDC defines occupational HIV exposure as percutaneous injury with a contaminated sharp or exposure of non-intact skin or mucous membranes to infectious material, such as blood or body fluids. The transmission risk is 0.3% with sharps and 0.09% with other exposure. Prophylaxis is considered 80% effective based on limited studies. Exposure is classified in 3 ways:

- *Exposure material:* Blood or blood-contaminated fluids have established transmission while other body fluids, such as CSF, urine, stool, and tears or only theoretically or potentially infectious.
- *Exposure type:* a few drops of fluid are less contagious than a major splash, and a superficial or solid needle injury are less contagious than a large bore hollow needle with obvious blood contaminant or deep injury.
- *Exposure source:* asymptomatic HIV positive with viral load <1500 c/mL is a low risk, but symptomatic HIV positive, AIDS, acute retroviral syndrome, or viral load >1500 c/mL are high risks. Low risk is usually assumed if source cannot be tested.

Post-exposure prophylaxis (PEP) for HIV should be initiated as soon as possible within 24 hours even for suspected exposure and continued for 4 weeks. If the suspected source proves to be HIV negative, then PEP can be discontinued:

- Low-risk exposure: usually treated with a 2-drug protocol.
- High-risk exposure: usually treated with a $\geq$ 3-drug protocol.

The HCW should be re-evaluated at 72 hours, and HIV serology tests should be done initially to establish a baseline, at 6 weeks, 12 weeks and 6 months. If there is HCV seroconversion, then HIV serology must be done at 12 months as well. Monitoring must be done for evidence of toxicity related to treatment while PEP is administered. Seroconversions must be reported according to guidelines to public health officials. HCWs receiving PEP should be counseled regarding secondary transmission of the virus to others and provided with information about safe sex practices.

HBV

Hepatitis B (HBV) is highly contagious through blood and body fluids and is easily transmissible through a sharps injury, but transmission has been recorded in HCWs without sharp injuries from exposure of mucous membranes or non-intact skin to infective material. HBV in dried blood on environmental surfaces can remain viable for one week. Previously vaccinated adults are usually not tested, but HCWs with occupational exposure may be tested to determine serologic response and may be administered additional vaccine. Exposure to blood products that have both positive surface antigens (HBsAg) and e antigens (HbeAG) causes increased risk of infection. HBV post-exposure prophylaxis (PEP) is effective if administered within 24 hours. A combination of passive HB immunoglobulin (HBIG) and active HB vaccination may be used for PEP or a series of vaccinations alone. HCWs who have documented completion of HBV vaccination series but have not had post-vaccination serology should be given a booster.

HCV

Hepatitis C virus (HCV) is not efficiently transmitted through contact with blood contact with mucous membranes or non-intact skin and has been linked only to sharps injury with hollow-bore needles. Follow-up serology after exposure should be done to determine if there has been transmission of HCV so that early diagnosis and referral can be made. The risk of environmental contamination appears to be very low. There is no post-exposure prophylaxis that has proven effective at this time. Those who convert to seropositive for HCV should receive counselling in a number of areas:
- Liver protection: People who are positive should avoid alcohol, non-prescription drugs or prescription drugs that may damage the liver.
- Transmission risk: People should not donate blood or tissue and should cover cuts or sores to avoid spreading infection.
- Evaluation for chronic liver disease: People should have liver function tests.

SARS-CoV

Severe acute respiratory syndrome corona virus (SARS-CoV), first identified in 2002. SARS is highly contagious through airborne means and may present as a case of flu with fever and chills but rapidly causes pneumonia or acute respiratory distress syndrome. Isolation and barrier precautions are adequate protection, but diagnosis may be delayed, posing a threat to family, healthcare workers, and other patients. Staff who have had high-risk exposure, such as to being present in an aerosol-generating procedure, to SARS should be restricted from work and advised to stay at home and avoid contact with others for at least 10 days, the usual incubation time, with vigilant monitoring of fever and signs of respiratory infection with guidance from public health officials. Staff with low-risk exposure, such as contact without adequate barrier protection but without aerosol contamination can continue to work with temperatures taken BID and vigilant monitoring or respiratory symptoms.

Tuberculosis and the booster phenomeno

Tuberculosis testing often involves skin testing with the PPD test. A two-step procedure is now recommended because of the possibility of false negatives and to prevent misdiagnosis on the basis of the booster phenomenon.

A negative PPD finding can occur with an old infection because sensitivity wanes over time; however, subsequent tests months later might react positively because of the "boost" caused by the first test, suggesting an acute or recent infection and leading to unnecessary treatment. Therefore, with the two-step procedure, a second test is done 1-3 weeks after the first to determine the effect of the first test. If the second test converts to positive in this short period of time, then it is considered evidence of a boosted reaction to a previous infection. If the second test is negative, it is considered a true negative and subsequent changes to positive would be considered new infections.

Exposure to tuberculosis (TB) in a healthcare facility is almost always the result of inadequate or delayed diagnosis of active TB in a patient. Upon diagnosis, immediate contact investigation must be done to determine all those who might be at risk of infection, including nursing, laboratory, and housekeeping staff. A two-step PPD skin testing or the QuantiFERON®-TB Gold test should be done to determine if those exposed have become infected. Those who test positive must be evaluated to ensure that they do not have active TB. Treatment protocols for latent or active TB must be initiated as soon as possible. There are a number of different protocols, but for latent TB Isoniazid (INH) for 9 months is the treatment of choice. Healthcare workers with active pulmonary or laryngeal TB or who stopped treatment must be excluded from work until symptoms subside and 3 sputum tests are negative or treatment is completed.

Needlestick injuries
Needlestick injuries are the most common type of exposure experienced by health care workers providing direct patient care as well as housekeeping staff or environmental services workers who may come in contact with contaminated needles. It is estimated that there are 600,000 to 800,000 needlestick injuries annually, and it is required that they be reported, but the reality is that surveys have indicated that only about 1/5th of injuries are reported for a variety of reasons, such as staff being too busy, being embarrassed, or being unconcerned because the injury did not appear to break the skin. Most injuries are related to the use of syringes even with safety devices. A program to investigate and follow-up needlestick injuries must include a concerted campaign to educate staff on the importance of reporting injuries so that accurate baseline data can be obtained and evaluations of the injuries with necessary interventions can be done.

Emergency-response personnel exposed to communicable disease

First responders, such as police, firefighters, and emergency medical technicians may be exposed to communicable diseases before a diagnosis is made or may not be informed of a diagnosis, so the ICP must have a program in place to monitor, inform, and follow-up exposures. All first responder groups should be identified and a notification system devised, including information about contact persons and healthcare providers for the first responders. When a communicable disease is diagnosed, a contact investigation should include first responders as well as facility staff. Contact should be made immediately by telephone and in writing, especially important if post-exposure prophylaxis is needed. The ICP should be the designated contact person at the facility if first responders need to report communicable diseases that might have infected patients on the way to the facility. The ICP should coordinate any testing of source patients or providing information that may be necessary to treat exposure in first responders.

Analysis and trending of occupational exposure incidents

Occupational exposure incidents are a major area of concern for any facility. Needlestick injuries are the most common, with an estimated 600,000 to 800,000 annually in the United States, many going unreported. Other incidents may include accidental ingestion or skin contact. The infection control plan must clearly define occupational exposure incidents and part of the staff education must be the understanding that 100% of incidents must be reported immediately by the person involved in the incident or anyone observing the incident. An incident report form, print or electronic, must be available to all departments and staff. The ICP monitors all exposure incidents and gathers data about types of incidents and frequency, using analysis to determine if there is an increase or decrease. Monitoring trends in exposure is especially important if new safety measures, such as the use of needle safety devices, are instituted so that effectiveness can be determined.

Regulatory standards for occupational exposure to infectious material

OSHA requires that safeguards to prevent occupational exposure and incidents be a part of infection control policies. Additionally, the FDA has requirements related to the safety of medical devices. Some states have regulations that are more restrictive than those of OSHA. Important elements include:
- An exposure control plan that outlines methods to reduce staff injury/ exposure.
- Use of universal precautions at all times with all patients.
- Planning work practices to minimize danger and using newer and safer technologies as they become available, such as needles engineered to prevent injury.
- Sharps disposal methods that prohibit bending, recapping, shearing, breaking, or handling contaminated needles or other sharps. Scooping with one hand may be used if recapping is essential.
- Workers must be trained in use of universal precautions and methods to decrease exposure.
- Procedures for post-exposure evaluation and treatment must be part of exposure control plan.
- Immunization with Hepatitis B vaccine available to healthcare workers.

Immunization of staff

During seasonal outbreaks of influenza, staff may be infected in the community or by contact with infected patients. Prompt immunization of staff can help to curtail outbreaks as staff are commonly exposed and may spread infection to multiple patients if infected. The ICP should ensure that all staff, especially those with direct patient contact, receive annual influenza vaccinations. The CDC provides guidelines for immunization of both patients and staff who are not immunized. Those that apply to staff include the following:
- Rapid influenza virus testing for staff with recent onset of symptoms.
- Restricting staff movement from outbreak areas.
- dministering current season's vaccination to those not immunized.
- Providing influenza antiviral prophylaxis and treatment according to most current recommendations. Prophylaxis should be considered for all staff, even those immunized, if the influenza is a variant and not matched by the vaccine.
- Removing infected staff from direct patient care, especially in high-risk areas.

Surgery may be limited to emergency procedures and elective procedures postponed.

Work restriction

The level of work restriction for health care workers exposed to a communicable disease varies considerably according to the type of infection. Typical restrictions from work include:
- *Tuberculosis* requires restriction of those with active pulmonary or pharyngeal TB until they have had adequate treatment, symptoms subside, and 3 sputum cultures are negative.
- *Influenza* requires restriction 7 days after the onset of symptoms and should be restricted from duty.
- *Measles* requires restriction from 5 days after first exposure to 21 days after the last.
- *Mumps* requires restriction from the 12th day after exposure to the 26th day.
- *Rubella* requires restriction from the 7th day after exposure to the 21st.
- *Pertussis* requires restriction for the first 5 days of treatment after onset of symptoms.
- *Herpetic whitlow* (intense Herpes Simplex infection of the fingers) requires restriction until lesions heal as they may shed virus even with gloves.

Various types of symptoms pose the risk of being associated with infectious diseases and infection control policies should contain guidelines for immediately reporting these symptoms to employee health/infection control and applying work restrictions:

- Diarrhea can be related to infectious processes and any staff with diarrhea, especially those with direct patient contact or food workers, should be restricted from duty until symptoms clear.
- Skin rashes can be caused by viral diseases, such as chickenpox or measles, and workers should be restricted from duty according to diagnosis.
- Cough can be caused by viral or bacterial infections and staff should be evaluated and restricted from work until cough clears.
- Dermatitis, especially on the hands, should be evaluated for work restriction and causes, and treatment provided. If a latex allergy is causing the dermatitis, that could pose a serious risk to the staff person as well as leading to infection of irritated skin that can infect others.

Assessment of risk of occupational exposure

Part of the determination regarding screening and immunizations depends upon the risk of occupational exposure, and this may vary by job classification and from one department to another. This determination requires careful auditing of positions to determine which ones have direct patient contact that could result in transmission of infection. Staff may be at risk from airborne or droplet transmission even though they are not involved in direct patient care, including environmental and nutritional services staff who enter patient rooms. Ideally, all personnel employed in a healthcare facility would have the basic recommended vaccinations in order to reduce risk. A system should be in place to quickly identify anyone who has had contact with a patient later diagnosed with an infectious disease. All visits to patients' rooms by nursing, laboratory, physical therapy, environmental, respiratory, nutritional, or other services should be by assigned personnel with records maintained regarding contact.

Counseling

Providing counseling to health care workers exposed to a communicable disease is extremely important, especially those exposed to a serious disease, such as HIV or TB. The HCW may face the possibility of medications, side effects, debility, or even death. In some cases, infection might pose a risk to family members or negatively affect relationships. While people react differently to exposure incidents, studies have indicated that over 40% of staff that have exposure incidents report increased stress and depression after the event. Some have reported symptoms consistent with post-traumatic stress disorder (PTSD) with nightmares and panic attacks. Others have left the field of health care altogether as a result of exposure. The infection control plan should include plans for counseling for all staff involved in exposure incidents and automatic referrals should be mad with each event. A counselor should be provided free of charge or health care plans should provide for counseling.

Information exchange between employee health and infection control departments

Occupational/employee health and infection control departments must work closely together because employee health and exposure issues are in the purview of the ICP. In some facilities, the ICP is in charge of both areas, and in a small facility, this might be efficient, but only part of employee health issues relate to infection control, so this may not be the best utilization of expertise. The director of the employee health program and the ICP should attend each other's meetings when possible and should establish guidelines for the sharing of information so that both departments work cooperatively. While privacy issues are a matter of concern, staff should be provided with release forms that clearly state that all matters related to infection control would be shared between the departments. The infection control and employee health departments should collaborate on the development of policies, new employee orientation and infection control education.

Practice Test

Practice Questions

1. Which of the following statements regarding Clostridium difficile spores is NOT true?
    a. Hand washing is the most effective method to prevent C. difficile transmission.
    b. Spores are noninfectious forms of the organism.
    c. Ingestion triggers spore activation to their disease-causing form.
    d. Spores can be recovered from computer keyboards and window coverings.

2. Identify the TRUE statement regarding enterococcal infections in the United States:
    a. Most human enterococcal infections are due to Enterococcus avium.
    b. Enterococci are normal inhabitants of the gastrointestinal tract.
    c. Enterococci rarely show resistance to vancomycin.
    d. Gram stain typically reveals gram-negative diplococci in short chains.

3. Which of the following pathogens is the LEAST likely to be associated with nosocomial wound infections?
    a. Escherichia coli
    b. Staphylococcus aureus
    c. Coagulase-negative staphylococci
    d. Bacteroides fragilis

4. A hospital's infection control nurse reported postsurgical wound infections by classification in a group of patients. Which was classified correctly as clean-contaminated (class II)?
    a. Closed reduction of Colles fracture in 74-year-old woman
    b. Emergency appendectomy and abscess evacuation in febrile 18-year-old man
    c. Elective thoracotomy with right upper lobectomy in 52-year-old smoker
    d. Stab wound to abdomen with intestinal perforation in 25-year-old man

5. A comparison of the incidence of lung cancer in a population of smokers compared with the incidence in a nonsmoking population defines which statistical term?
    a. Relative risk
    b. Incidental risk
    c. Disease prevalence
    d. Disease incidence

6. A large community hospital's tumor registry reports a marked decrease in cases of hepatocellular carcinoma over a 20-year period. Which of the following is LEAST likely to account for this occurrence?
    a. Improved serologic screening of transfusion donors
    b. Higher vaccination rates for hepatitis A
    c. Higher community vaccination rates for hepatitis B
    d. Decreased prevalence of seropositivity for hepatitis C over same period

7. Match the following elements of outbreak case definitions with the appropriate examples:

1) Person   4) Clinical features
2) Place   5) Laboratory features
3) Time

a. Onset during winter months December through March, 2008
b. Sputum positive for acid-fast bacilli
c. Day-shift medical technologists at tertiary-care hospital
d. Allcare Rehabilitation, Yuma, Arizona
e. Morbilliform rash

8. World Health Organization 2009 published guidelines for hand hygiene include all of the following EXCEPT:

a. After cleansing and rinsing, use a towel to turn off spigot and do not re-use.
b. Use of warm or hot water for rinsing to kill off any remaining bacteria
c. Hand hygiene is needed after removing gloves used for wound dressings.
d. Use of soap and water if alcohol-based hand rubs are not available.

9. What percentage of nosocomial infections is believed to be caused by bacterial contamination carried by hands of caregivers and health care workers?

a. 50%
b. 33%
c. 25%
d. 15%

10. An intensive care unit (ICU) patient in a metropolitan hospital is diagnosed with culture-positive non-acid-fast multidrug resistant bacteria (MDR). This occurs 1 week after admission to the same ICU of a homeless 46-year-old man with pneumonia and underlying COPD who was also diagnosed with MDR. Infection control surveillance should include all of the following EXCEPT:

a. Masks for patient and all caregivers
b. Strict handwashing precautions
c. Decontamination procedures for all portable chest radiography
d. Surface culture samples of shared diagnostic or invasive equipment

11. A pathogen that appears to be transmitted by airborne spread is suspected in an outbreak affecting a heavily ethnic section of a metropolitan area. Important initial public communications strategies should include:

a. Early announcements with tempered reassurances
b. Delayed announcements until all information is gathered
c. Adherence to the "decide and announce" model
d. Disregard for culturally based interpretations in favor of rational explanations

12. Proper transport protocol for blood samples drawn from an acutely ill homosexual man admitted with to the ICU with acute pneumonia and unknown serologic status for HIV requires:

a. Single-compartment waterproof packaging with surrounding absorbent material
b. Double-layer waterproof packaging, absorbent material
c. Double-layer waterproof packaging, absorbent material, and appropriate documentation
d. Double-layer waterproof packaging, absorbent material, and appropriate documentation enclosed by outer packaging

13. Infectivity risks for transmission of HIV from patients to health care workers:
    a. Are highest with encounters involving needles and sharps.
    b. Occur at about the same rate as transmission of hepatitis b given similar direct exposures.
    c. Are often associated with asymptomatic carriers of hiv.
    d. A and c only

14. Identification of Bacillus anthracis:
    a. Shows gram-positive diplococci in short chains.
    b. Shows gram-negative diplococci in short chains.
    c. Shows gram-positive nonmotile rods.
    d. Requires immediate quarantine precautions of index case.

15. Diseases caused by arboviruses:
    a. Are only associated with overt clinical symptoms and syndromes in humans.
    b. Include dengue and yellow fever.
    c. Typically involve high rates of human-to-human transmission.
    d. Are more frequent in winter in the united states.

16. With regard to communicable diseases, the term contamination:
    a. Always implies a carrier state.
    b. Includes noninfectious environmental pollutants.
    c. Describes infectious particles on body surfaces and inanimate objects.
    d. Does not apply to infectious agents in foods and liquids.

Questions 17 through 19 pertain to the following clinical case:
    An athletic 32-year-old man is admitted with fever and convulsive episodes that have rendered him comatose. History obtained from his wife includes a prodrome of headaches and hydrophobia. She recalls he had complained about tingling around an area that had been affected by a small right shoulder wound a couple of weeks ago. She says that he had otherwise been well since his return from China 1 month ago on an adventure vacation that included visits to bat-infested caves and rural farms. She reports they have a cat and two dogs at home, all in usual apparent health. Routine blood and cerebrospinal fluid have been drawn for cell counts, cultures, and any ancillary testing.

17. Diagnostic work-up should also immediately prioritize:
    a. Saliva or skin testing for rabies virus nucleic acid amplification by reverse transcriptase polymerase chain reaction (RT-PCR).
    b. Brain biopsy to submit tissue for mouse cell culture at reference laboratory.
    c. Brain biopsy to identify toxoplasma cysts.
    d. Blood and CSF culture for rabies using vitamin-enhanced media

18. The incubation period for the primary diagnosis under consideration:
    a. Is within a week following ingestion of undercooked, infected meat.
    b. Is highly variable but often occurs within 3 to 8 weeks after exposure.
    c. Does not appear to be related to location of wound or protective clothing.
    d. Has a typical duration of 1 to 3 days.

19. Appropriate infection control measures should include:
   a. Quarantine of index case
   b. Formal report to local health authorities
   c. Postexposure prophylaxis of intimate, mucous-membrane contacts with immune globulin
   d. B and C

20. A male health care worker from the Philippines who is applying for a surgery scrub tech position tests positive for hepatitis B surface antibody, negative for hepatitis B e antigen (HBeAg), and negative for hepatitis B surface antigen (HBsAg). Which is the best interpretation or recommendation in light of these findings?
   a. He is likely immunized to hepatitis B by prior vaccination.
   b. He is likely to have chronic hepatitis B infection.
   c. He is likely to be a carrier and should not be offered the surgical suite position.
   d. He is likely to be highly infectious and should receive hepatitis B immune globulin.

21. Which of the following statements regarding normal flora in humans is NOT true?
   a. Normal flora may be further classified into resident and transient flora.
   b. By definition, colonization by normal flora does not result in infection.
   c. Normal flora contains commensal microbes that are neither harmful nor beneficial to the host.
   d. Normal flora may participate in nutrient synthesis or excretion.

22. Preliminary throat cultures from an 83-year-old nursing home resident are reported to you as "positive for beta-hemolytic streptococci." You are aware of two other residents of the same nursing home with new-onset fever and exudative pharyngitis this week. Initial surveillance and investigation entails all of the following EXCEPT:
   a. Immunization of visitors and health care personnel in contact with index cases.
   b. Ensure rapid antigen detection methods are available and properly used and reported by nursing home personnel.
   c. Isolation of index cases with staff education and implementation of precautions involving secretions and drainage.
   d. Investigate possible outbreak sources from possible contacts, carriers, and food contamination (milk, milk products).

23. Which of the following characterizes syndromic surveillance methodology in outbreak detection?
   a. Low sensitivity and high specificity of case definitions
   b. Rapid detection of outbreaks based on clinical diagnoses evidenced by laboratory findings
   c. Fixed parameters of suspect case definitions over time
   d. Employs broad general descriptive terms (e.g., influenza-like symptoms) and short-term statistical analysis

24. The incubation period of a transmissible disease:
   a. Is the time period between invasion by a pathogenic microbe and initial signs of altered tissue status or infection onset.
   b. Is not defined for situations in which the host organism is a vector.
   c. Occurs between a narrow window of days to weeks.
   d. Is independent of variations in host resistance and environmental factors.

Categorize the following uses of antimicrobials using the three patient scenarios below, in the order given below to answer Question 25:

Patient A is brought to the surgical suite for elective hip replacement surgery is administered an anti-infective agent active against skin flora.

Patient B begins oral antimalarials prior to travel to an endemic area.

Patient C is a kidney-transplant recipient admitted for suspected rejection. An antifungal is ordered for oral thrush noted on initial exam.

25. The categorization of the uses of antimicrobials using the three patient scenarios above in the order given above are:
    a. Empiric, prophylactic, therapeutic
    b. Prophylactic, empiric, therapeutic
    c. Therapeutic, empiric, prophylactic
    d. Prophylactic, prophylactic, therapeutic

26. Nosocomial infections include all of the following EXCEPT:
    a. Postsurgical wound infection identified in outpatient suture clinic 1 week following hospital discharge.
    b. Neonatal herpes diagnosed in newborn infant vaginally delivered from HSV-infected mother.
    c. Congenital malformations in newborn with positive IgM titer for rubella.
    d. Diagnosis of nosocomial infection made by attending surgeon.

27. A new infection control nurse seeks to revamp the infection surveillance system of a 125-patient bed community hospital. The hospital information system's (HIS) technology is old yet is highly utilized by medical staff and health care personnel. Which assessment is most accurate?
    a. Passive surveillance that relies upon reporting by health care personnel and laboratory data is likely to capture and correctly classify most data.
    b. Active surveillance is likely to be more expensive and require more manpower but is likely to yield accurate and more comprehensive data.
    c. Laboratory-based plans are likely to succeed in an acceptable HIS setting, regardless of whether specific disease-monitoring protocols are in place.
    d. Patient-based plans should prove more time-efficient and cost-effective compared with laboratory-based plans.

28. All of the following statements regarding postdischarge surveillance of hospitalized patients is true EXCEPT:
    a. Most hospitals follow standardized postdischarge surveillance guidelines.
    b. Decreased length of stay impedes capture of postsurgical wound infection rates.
    c. Telephone interviews or mailed questionnaires are two methods that can be successfully employed.
    d. Postdischarge follow-up via physician office records may be incomplete or not timely.

29. The T-point classification system:
   a. Is one method of assessing risk of postoperative infection in surgical patients
   b. Examines multiple variables used in assessing risk of surgical infection
   c. Assigns a percentile time score based on average hours a surgical procedure is performed at the index hospital
   d. Indicates a lower risk for infection when t points are exceeded

30. The 0 to 3 point scoring system using the CDC National Nosocomial Infections Surveillance (NNIS) Risk Index:
   a. Assigns a score of -1 (minus 1) for no risk factors
   b. Assigns 1 point for clean-contaminated surgical cases.
   c. Assigns 2 points for exceeding a surgical procedure's t point
   d. Assigns 1 point for preoperative american society of anesthesiologists (asa) scores of 3 to 5

Answer questions 31 and 32 based on the following information:

A hospital seeks to assess its overall central line infection rate. You are asked to report overall infection rates using device days based on the following data obtained:

Service	# of Patients	Total # Device Days	Total # Infections
Medical intensive care unit	12	48	2
Surgical intensive care unit	9	20	1
Oncology ward	15	72	4

31. Based on these data, the overall hospital central line infection rate per 1,000 device days is:
   a. 5
   b. 7
   c. 50
   d. 257

32. Based on device days, the service with the highest infection rate is:
   a. Medical intensive care unit
   b. Surgical intensive care unit
   c. Surgical intensive care unit, but not statistically significant
   d. Oncology ward

33. Which of the following data sets is MOST likely to meet statistical significance?
   a. P value < 0.05 in study of 7 patients with uncomplicated seasonal influenza
   b. P value < 0.05 in study of 100 patients with complicated seasonal influenza
   c. P value > 0.05 in study of 1,000 patients with complicated seasonal influenza
   d. P value > 0.05 in study of 1,000 patients with uncomplicated seasonal influenza

34. Agents and methods used to sterilize or disinfect are segregated into three tiers. Which of the following statement is NOT accurate regarding these categories?
   a. Low-level agents, such as iodophors, kill most bacteria and fungi, but not viruses.
   b. Alcohol is an intermediate disinfectant that does not kill or inactivate spores.
   c. Hydrogen peroxide is an example of a high-level disinfectant.
   d. High disinfectants may not eradicate high concentrations of bacterial spores.

35. Methods of flash sterilization:
    a. Employ temperatures of at least 132°C for 10 minutes or less
    b. Are not recommended for surgical equipment meant for re-use
    c. Involves dry heat using oven-type equipment for as long as needed
    d. Will not kill vegetative organisms or viruses, even when items are precleaned.

36. Decubiti in spinal cord injury patients:
    a. Are not commonly associated with spread of infection to nearby bone
    b. Typically show single, dominant organisms on culture
    c. Occur in about two-thirds of patients with such neurologic injuries
    d. Are related to pressure and contamination

37. Which of the following actions is NOT considered an effective infection control strategy in surgical environments?
    a. Preferential use of flash sterilization
    b. 15 or more air exchanges hourly
    c. Hallways and nearby areas ventilated with positive pressure
    d. Wet-vacuum mechanical cleaning of surgical suites at end of day

38. The role of nutritional services in a hospital's overall infection control program:
    a. Necessitates use of disposable materials, such as paper napkins, plates, and utensils
    b. Requires delivery staff to move items such as bedpans aside so food tray can be deposited
    c. Requires health care personnel to deliver trays to patients on airborne precautions
    d. Includes removal of food trays contaminated by body fluids provided nutritional orderly cleanses area immediately

39. In order to comply with the Safe Medical Devices Act of 1990, medical facilities that use medical devices associated with complications such as injury or death:
    a. Must report incidents requiring medical or surgical intervention within 48 hours
    b. Must file semiannual and annual medical device reporting (mdr)
    c. May use medwatch forms as needed without need for written procedures
    d. Must retain records related to medical device reports for 10 years

40. While assisting in paracentesis of a patient with chronic liver failure, an emergency department nurse's aide reports a splash incident and claims he felt a drop of ascitic fluid hit his eye. According to required elements in the hospital's exposure control plan, which of the following steps must be followed?
    a. Immediate postexposure prophylaxis with hepatitis B immune globulin (HBIG).
    b. Identify staff member and exposure incident to rest of hospital staff.
    c. Cease all paracentesis procedures in ED until investigation is complete.
    d. Review OSHA standards for procedure and document event compliance.

41. An announcement in the hospital newsletter about a hand washing contest that involves a special glow-in-the-dark powder is MOST likely:
    a. A hands-on method of promoting infection control practices to staff.
    b. A waste of valuable health care worker time.
    c. An educational opportunity that will only benefit students.
    d. Less effective than posters that show proper hand washing technique.

42. An infection control program's annual summary:
   a. Does not need to be filed if no incidents occurred
   b. Is a document whose purpose is to summarize occupational exposures
   c. Is a budgetary document used to determine cost-benefit ratios
   d. Documents adherence to infection control program's goals specific to outcomes and objectives

43. As the first dedicated infection control officer hired at a new hospital, what initial assessments should you make in designing your institution's infection control plan?
   a. Determine patient population, institutional size, services, and departments
   b. Request funding to hire IT consultants to upgrade hardware and software
   c. Develop 30-day client satisfaction survey regarding infection control plan
   d. Perform cost-benefit analysis of most frequently performed procedures

44. CDC recommendations regarding appropriate nail care for health care personnel whose duties include direct patient care or contact with food and supplies include:
   a. Trimming nails to one-quarter inch length
   b. Routine cultures of subungual areas of artificial nails or nail tip.
   c. Allowance of artificial nails or tips of any length with fresh polish applied daily
   d. Routine use of double-thickness gloves for artificial-nail wearers

45. The power to issue recalls and regulations regarding reuse issues involving medications and medical devices is held by the:
   a. Occupational Safety and Health Administration
   b. The Joint Commission
   c. Food and Drug Administration
   d. Centers for Disease Control and Prevention

46. The Shewhart cycle refers to:
   a. A circular diagram used to analyze cause and effect
   b. A quality management tool for problem-solving
   c. A type of pareto charting
   d. A schematic flow chart

47. While at lunch in the hospital cafeteria, you hear a group of nurses talking about how it seems as though every child whose urinary catheter was inserted in the emergency department develops a UTI. Your educational planning includes a series of in-service talks with PowerPoint presentations and handouts. To maximize effectiveness:
   a. Handouts are delivered by speaker as s/he begins presentation.
   b. Handouts should be lengthy and use large blocks of text.
   c. Handouts should be legible copy of powerpoint presentation.
   d. Handouts should highlight the presentation's key points.

48. The departments of anesthesiology and surgery seek to work with infection control to increase perioperative antibiotic use within 30 minutes of skin incision. Your approach includes all of the following EXCEPT:

    a. Calculate compliance as number of surgical procedures divided by number of times antibiotic is given within 30 minutes of incision.

    b. Identify behaviors that may contribute to delay or omission of delivering antibiotic within 30 minutes of incision.

    c. Demonstrate appropriate perioperative time management, reinforce correct timing of dose, and monitor until desired behaviors are satisfactorily adopted.

    d. Use before and after data analysis of surgical infection rates as surrogate or observational marker of compliance.

49. Which of the following recommended procedures regarding pre-employment vetting of health care workers is required by the Joint Commission?

    a. Testing for drugs of abuse and background check

    b. Tuberculin skin testing (purified protein derivative [PPD])

    c. Chest radiograph for positive PPD results

    d. Vaccination against hepatitis B for nonimmune candidates

50. Which of the following health care workers who are normally involved in direct patient care should be placed on work restriction?

    a. Skin rash following course of amoxicillin for otitis media

    b. Latex glove skin allergy by history with no active lesions

    c. Small finger lesion consistent with herpetic whitlow

    d. New-onset nonproductive cough in nurse on ACE inhibitor antihypertensive

Answers and Explanations

1. A: In a manner similar to the spores of Bacillus anthracis, an outermost layer of Clostridium difficile spores called the exosporium renders these microbes sticky, which enables them to adhere to health care workers' hands or environmental surfaces, such as computer keyboards, window coverings, and telephones, used by clinical staff. The most effective prevention strategy is barrier protection, as in rigorous adherence to glove use, which should always be followed by thorough hand washing. Although many commercial products claim to rid hands of spores, their success rates are less than that of barrier methods. Spores are the noninfectious forms of the organisms, which are activated following ingestion to their disease-causing form.

2. B: The ubiquity and increasing antimicrobial resistance patterns among Enterococcus spp. is an infection control challenge for health care facilities worldwide. Vancomycin-resistant strains are frequently reported in the United States. These enteric, facultative gram-positive cocci grow in short chains. They are normal inhabitants of the gastrointestinal tract (large bowel) and female genitourinary tract. While E. faecalis causes the majority of infections and shows emerging resistance to many antibiotics, E. faecium isolates demonstrate a high degree of vancomycin resistance. Because many nosocomial enterococcal infections are transmitted by contact, these organisms are also found on skin and wounds, often as a result of hand carriage by health care workers.

3. D: The bacterial species most commonly responsible for surgical site infections (SSI) is Staphylococcus aureus. In one study, this species accounted for 20% of all SSI. Given this microbe's increasing rates of antimicrobial resistance, as in methicillin-resistant S. aureus (MRSA), these infections represent a formidable foe in terms of mortality, morbidity, and increasing health care costs. Following S. aureus in frequency are those infections caused by coagulase-negative staphylococci (14%), as in S. epidermidis, frequently found on skin and mucous membranes as normal bacterial flora. These organisms are often associated with infections related to indwelling devices and catheters, and in endocarditis. Following staphylococci in frequency are wound infections involving enterococcus (12%) and E. coli (8%). Although infections involving anaerobic Bacteroides fragilis are worrisome, these organisms accounted for only 2% of all SSI in the study noted, following other more frequently occurring infections related to pathogens such as Pseudomonas, Klebsiella, Proteus, and Enterobacter species.

4. C: Clean-contaminated or class II surgical wounds may involve entry into parts of the body that normally contain flora, such as the respiratory or urinary tracts; however, in order to qualify as class II, such procedures must be elective and not violate aseptic technique nor show evidence of an infectious process. By definition, the closed wrist fracture reduction does not involve a break in skin and would be a class I procedure. The emergency appendectomy with evidence of abscess implicates perforation and infection, and is thus a class IV wound. The elective thoracotomy with right upper lobe resection involves the respiratory tract, a potential source of contamination. However, surgery was elective and did not note infection or break in technique, so it is correctly classified as clean-contaminated.

5. A: Relative risk (RR) is a useful statistical term in infectious epidemiology as well as noninfectious disease surveillance. Although a noninfectious example is used here, the concept remains important to understanding risk of disease transmission in certain populations. Relative risk is a ratio that shows the risk of developing a disease or infection in a population exposed to a causative agent compared with the risk for developing the same entity in a population that is not exposed to that agent. Because RR involves two ratios, that of the event probability in the exposed group divided by that in the unexposed group, it is also known as the risk ratio. Disease prevalence references the number of cases of a disease in a given population at a set time; disease incidence represents the frequency or rate at which new

cases of a disease are seen in a given population during a specified time frame. Disease incidence is often used in epidemiologic investigations.

6. B: The greatest risk factor for the development of hepatocellular carcinoma (hepatoma) worldwide is infectious. Hepatitis B is a viral infection endemic in much of the non-Western world for which an effective vaccine has been available since the 1980s. Hepatitis A, for which there is also an effective vaccine delivered in two doses spaced 6 to 12 months apart, does not show strong statistical correlation with development of hepatocellular carcinoma, in contrast to data involving hepatitis B and C viruses. Twinrix, a vaccination against both hepatitis A and B, is administered in three doses, similar to that given against hepatitis B alone. Increased rates of hepatocellular carcinoma in Western countries has paralleled increased rates of hepatitis C, and appear likely due to increased use of blood products, growing populations of intravenous drug users, and chronicity of infections caused by hepatitis C–tainted blood products administered in the past. Serologic screening improvements have helped decrease the number of transfusion-associated nosocomial infections caused by these viruses.

7. 1-C, 2-D, 3-A, 4-E, 5-B. Essential data that must be collected during the investigation of an outbreak reference person, place, time of event, and its clinical and laboratory features. In this match, the person can represent a defined group as in the day-shift technologists of choice C. The place is the facility in Arizona. The time can be a reference period, as in the winter months of choice A. Clinical features include signs and symptoms, as in the morbilliform rash of choice E, and other clinical findings or comments regarding disease transmission. Laboratory features include those diagnostic findings such as results of cultures, special serology, or specialized testing as in polymerase chain reaction (PCR), immunofixation, or other techniques that specify the nature of the infection.

8. B: Hand hygiene remains an opportunity area for increased compliance and improved technique. Warm or hot water is not recommended for rinsing off soap or other disinfectant materials because of the increased risk for skin irritation or dermatitis that may be caused by higher water temperatures combined with topical chemicals. Rather, use of a towel or disposable napkin is recommended following cleansing before handling spigots or other community-soiled areas with prompt disposal of said item, not to be reused again. Even use of gloves is not fail-safe. In fact, hand washing is recommended after gloves are removed as in the wound-dressing example here. Alcohol-based hand rubs are effective when used around all surfaces of hands and fingers until dry; however, soap and water can be effective when such agents are not available.

9. D: Many studies attribute about 15% of nosocomial infections to contamination caused by hand carriage of pathogens by health care workers. These incidents may occur via direct patient-to-patient contact or with intermediary static objects that may be contact-contaminated, from computer keyboards, pens, or even radiologic equipment. The latter is a common occurrence in ICU settings where portable radiography is employed. Many health care workers erroneously believe (or become complacent through years of clinical practice) that the use of gloves trumps the need for meticulous hand hygiene, or do not understand or follow the need for proper hand washing even after gloves are removed. Particularly in settings where gloved health care workers come into contact with potentially devastating pathogens (e.g., C. difficile, antibiotic-resistant strains, MRSA), it is imperative that hand washing and other infection-control strategies be ingrained in staff, with appropriate reminders, surveillance, and continuing education as necessary.

10. A: Cross-contamination or cross-colonization may occur even with strict infection control precautions in place. Laxity in adhering to IC guidelines increases the likelihood of breaching IC standards, which may be especially hazardous with multidrug resistant organisms, particularly those that require long periods of complex antimicrobial therapy, as in multidrug-resistant tuberculosis

(MDR-TB). With isolation of a non-acid-fast organism, contact transmission appears more likely than airborne transmission that would indicate mask precautions for patient and caregivers. Surface cultures of shared equipment may help isolate the infectious culprit while rigorous decontamination procedures may halt the spread of infection to new unit admissions. As in any outbreak occurrence, increased vigilance to hand washing techniques should be enforced because suboptimal compliance by health care workers in multiple settings is frequently reported.

11. A: Transparency is at the core of effective communications strategies during outbreaks, which promotes trust among the public and aids in acceptance of the information conveyed. Even when all information has not been gathered and analyzed, early announcements are appropriate and may be tempered by accurate reassurances as more information emerges or recommendations shift. Communication delays until all information is known not only hinders trust but may increase public fear. Such delays also appear to show lack of leadership or inhibit outbreak containment. Failures of the expert-centered "decide and announce" model have caused strategists to largely abandon this one-way method. Instead, successful communications have shifted towards listening to public concerns, including cultural considerations, and a more open, two-way dialogue guided by organized operational planning.

12. D: The sample described fulfills criteria for a category A specimen, one that has the potential to cause permanent disability, life-threatening morbidity or death in immunologically intact, otherwise healthy humans or animals because of infectious agents the specimen may harbor. Proper transport for category A specimens dictates use of triple packaging as described in option D. In addition, packaging must be documented as having met performance criteria whereby adequate resistance has been shown to stresses by gravity, puncture, and pressure. Enclosed absorbent material must be of sufficient volume and absorbance capacity to take up all escaped fluids should breakage occur.

13. D: Even with improved infection control practices and heightened awareness, transmission of HIV from patients to health care workers remains an area of concern. The highest risk for exposure occurs in settings involving sharps and needles. Although there is a higher chance of knowing the HIV serologic status of patients today than in the past, there is a greater risk of infectivity of HIV to health care workers from patients with unknown or uncertain serologic status. Given similar exposures, the rate of seroconversion following exposure to infectious hepatitis B particles in the health care setting is about 25%, much greater than the 0.5% seroconversion rate for HIV. Such statistics underscore the need for a robust program of hepatitis B vaccination for health care workers and strict precautions in settings where hepatitis B is likely to occur, as in hospital populations from endemic areas, those with large numbers of intravenous drug abusers, dialysis units, and in endemic areas abroad.

14. C: Infection control personnel are often the first individuals notified of preliminary results, particularly when there is a high index of suspicion for a worrisome pathogen or one that involves a patient with an aggressive clinical course. IC staff must have working familiarity with the ways in which preliminary results are communicated, and understand differential diagnostic considerations and implications for action. Laboratories report results of preliminary gram-stain results, some of which help narrow diagnostic possibilities, as in the typical "tennis racket" appearance of Clostridium tetani, the infectious agent of tetanus. Here, Bacillus anthracis is a gram-positive rod associated with environmental flora in settings that involve livestock, such as sheep and cattle. Because it is transmitted via inhalation or breaks in intact skin or mucous membranes, quarantine precautions of the index are not indicated, while further investigations are certainly warranted.

15. B: Viruses are classified by many characteristics that may include their ribonucleic acid (DNA vs RNA), protein coat structure, virus size or shape, envelope coating (if any), and method of replication. Arboviruses are a taxonomic class of viruses that involve transmission by an arthropod insect vector

that is required for human infection to occur. The prototypical arboviral infection is malaria, spread by vector transmission by the Plasmodium falciparum mosquito species. Mosquitoes and ticks are common arbovirus vectors. Arboviruses are capable of causing acute and chronic infections; however, most acute infections are asymptomatic. In the case of malaria, disease may not manifest until a decade or more following initial exposure in extreme cases. Human-to-human transmission is not a factor in spread of these diseases. The vector of the dengue fever flavivirus is the Aedes aegypti mosquito; Aedes spp. mosquitoes also harbor the yellow fever flavivirus. In the Northern hemisphere, most cases of arboviral-associated encephalitis are reported in the warmer months, typically June through September.

16. C: Contamination is a term whose nuanced meanings must be thoroughly understood and properly communicated by infection control personnel. While a disease carrier may be contaminated by an infectious agent, the converse is not true and, therefore, contamination does not necessarily imply a carrier state. Materials that are considered contaminated by infectious agents include foods, liquids such as water or milk, or objects/substances that may harbor infectious agents on their surfaces or that may contain the infectious particles. These latter categories can include contaminated toys, bedding, or even items commonly found in health care settings such as surgical supplies. Noninfectious environmental pollutants are not considered contaminants for the purpose of infection control monitoring and surveillance, even though they may be irritating, offensive, or even noxious.

17. A: Symptoms of hydrophobia, headaches, and altered mental state progressing to coma should alert clinicians to rabies, particularly following travel to an endemic area and a history of a wound with paresthesias. Bites or scratches involving rabid animals closer to the head and neck area are of particular concern and may shorten the incubation period to disease manifestation. Choices B and C are unsuitable as brain biopsy is not an immediate diagnostic test choice but useful as postmortem confirmation. Rather, saliva or skin, especially the latter sampled from the hairline of the posterior neck region, may be tested by fluorescent antibody or RT-PCR for rabies. Cultures are not indicated for this viral disease. China has seen increased numbers of confirmed rabies cases, while rabies has decreased in other parts of Asia, particularly in Thailand.

18. B: The primary diagnosis under consideration is rabies, a disease in which the incubation period may vary depending on factors such as the proximity of the bite or scratch to the head and neck area; the depth of the wound; infectivity of the index animal; the virulence and concentration of virus delivered into the wound; and amount of protection offered by clothing or other protective coverings, such as backpacks. Because of these and other animal vector and host factors, the incubation period may fall between a few days or many years. Many rabies cases occur following incubation periods of 3 to 8 weeks. Choice A does not relate to the disease in question, nor would these symptoms appear typical for acute infection with toxoplasma, which is more typically asymptomatic or presents with a viral-type illness that might suggest infectious mononucleosis rather than the cataclysmic events in this case.

19. D: Quarantine of the human index case is not an appropriate action for suspected rabies as the incidence of person-to-person transmission is exceedingly rare, particularly in a controlled hospital setting. Rather, had this patient been bitten by a dog, cat, or other animal that remained in contact with humans, it would be appropriate to quarantine and observe the animal, perform appropriate diagnostic tests, and euthanize it as indicated. A formal report to local health authorities is required, and is likewise obligatory in many countries worldwide. In an attempt to neutralize viral load, efforts should be made to deliver passive prophylaxis with rabies immune globulin (human or equine) as soon as possible after the rabid attack. In addition, close contacts of the infected patient who have had mucous membrane exposure to the index case should also receive postexposure prophylaxis with immune globulin.

20. A: Following completion of the full, three-dose immunization schedule for hepatitis B, immune-competent vaccine recipients will show positive results for hepatitis B surface antibody but will have negative serology for the markers of current or past hepatitis B infection. HBeAg positivity is associated with a high degree of potential infectivity while positive results for hepatitis B surface antigen (HBsAg) indicate a potentially infectious carrier state. HBsAg may be detected any time within a wide time frame, from initial acute infection to years later when the disease enters a chronic phase. The chronic active carrier state for hepatitis B would be expected to show positive serologic markers for HBsAg and HBcAb. The diagnosis of chronic hepatitis requires additional marker seropositivity, elevation of liver enzymes, biopsy confirmation, or other ancillary studies.

21. B: Up to a thousand different microbial species live on or inside our bodies. Because these microbes do not normally cause disease or infections, they are termed normal flora. Some normal flora is present at all times while the presence of other transient microbes ebbs and flows. As normal flora multiply, the expanded microbial population colonizes the host, provided they remain nonpathogenic and do not invade tissues or cause infections or disease. However, in cases of immune compromise, colonizing organisms can take advantage of host defense weaknesses to cause disease as pathogens, which can result in infections. Commensal organisms that neither benefit nor harm the host organism also represent subsets of normal flora. Some normal flora function to mutual benefit, such as E. coli that feed off contents of their intestinal tract home, and where they benefit the host organism through their actions in nutrient synthesis (e.g., Vitamin K) or elimination.

22. A: In the laboratory, group A streptococci cause a visible clear zone of beta-hemolysis on sheep's blood agar culture plates. Group A strep are causative organisms in a wide variety of disease from sore ("strep") throat to the potentially lethal toxic shock syndrome (TSS). The organism is also capable of attacking heart valves, as in rheumatic heart disease that may ensue days or weeks following acute strep pharyngitis. There is no vaccine for group A streptococcal disease. All other steps B to D should be initiated while the outbreak is investigated. Milk and milk products have been identified in food-associated streptococcal outbreaks in which the food contamination is caused by transfer from humans infected with streptococci. Rapid antigen detection methods are handy and useful, provided they are made available in a timely fashion to staff and they are used and interpreted properly.

23. D: To investigate the source and scope of a potential outbreak, infection control professionals use syndromic surveillance to gather situational information and review broad clinical descriptions and impressions, rather than data from diagnostic testing. Because it acts as a large net, such surveillance should be designed for high sensitivity in order to capture data from as many patients who are actually positive for the disease in question. Low specificity is also desired, as specificity identifies the true negatives in such a study, such as patients who do not have a disease and their test results or assessment also shows that they do not appear to have the disease. Because parameters may need to be refined and adapted as more information is gathered, a surveillance system should also offer the flexibility to shift case definitions, clinical descriptors, such as "influenza-like symptoms," or other parameters over time.

24. A: An incubation period is defined as the time between invasion by a pathogenic microbe and initial signs of altered tissue status or onset of infection. When the host organism is a vector, the incubation period falls from vector invasion by the microbe to the next step in vector transmission, that is, when the vector spreads infection to other hosts, as in the bite of an infected mosquito. Diseases caused by some microbes involve longer incubation periods that may extend over years while other transmissible diseases can require mere hours before invasion is manifested as defined. Differences in incubation time length may be affected by variations in host factors, such as immune status, the virulence or type of

microbial pathogen, microbial load, and environmental factors, such as sanitation, pest control, and weather patterns.

25. D: Prophylactic antimicrobials are used to prevent infections before they occur. Although overuse of this preventive strategy has contributed to increased resistance to antimicrobials, evidence of its usefulness in many clinical scenarios is strong. One is in elective orthopedic reconstructive surgery, as in example A, wherein anti-infectives active against skin flora are typically used, often within 30 to 60 minutes of skin incision. Prophylaxis is also used with travel to areas of endemic illness, such as malaria, as in Patient B. Empiric antimicrobials are given when there is cause to suspect an infectious etiology but the specific microbe(s) has yet to be determined, as in a patient admitted with fever, cough, and purulent sputum. Patient C clinically shows oral thrush and is immune-suppressed. Therapeutic antimicrobials are given based on diagnosis, infective microbial identify, results of sensitivity tests as indicated, and relative cost factors. The clinical diagnosis of thrush in this case indicates therapeutic care. Routine culture and sensitivities are not generally performed in cases of this type.

26. C: Nosocomial infections encompass those hospital-acquired illness caused by pathogenic microbes that were not present in the index case when the patient entered the facility, whether the diagnosis is made during that stay or after discharge. Because infections categorized as nosocomial in nature may involve clinical as well as laboratory diagnoses, the diagnosis may also be made based on appropriate clinical data by an attending physician. The surgical site infection of Patient A occurred after discharge but is nosocomial in origin. The vaginal delivery in case B is the likely source of the neonate's herpes infection and is likewise nosocomial. However, the malformations and positive rubella titer in case C results from placental transfer of the rubella virus, which is not considered nosocomial.

27. B: Surveillance systems come in many types. When feasible, active surveillance is preferred over passive systems for completeness, accuracy, and consistency over time. Active programs require trained infection control staff and, thus, may be more costly. However, they are designed to root out hospital-acquired infections and involve proactive interventions. The accuracy and completeness of unmonitored passive systems rely upon reporting by health care personnel that may be incomplete or vary from one department to another. All plans, whether laboratory- or patient-based, require clear and well-constructed protocols to ensure timely and accurate reporting, regardless of the sophistication or version of HIS in place. Patient-based plans require more time for interviews and data collection and input, and therefore tend to be more costly than laboratory-based systems.

28. A: Decreased length of hospital stay may account for nearly half of missed cases of postdischarge, postoperative wound infections. Many different methods have been employed for postdischarge surveillance, in part because there is no standardized procedure that is universally accepted or that applies to the variety in health care settings, personnel, technology adaptation, and other factors. Telephone interviews, mailed questionnaires, and follow-up using physicians' postdischarge records and reports have all been used. The latter is prone to incompleteness and requires a dedicated effort to root out specific results that many office practices may not easily access, especially if the practice does not employ an efficient electronic health record system.

29. A: The T-point system is a method of assessing an institution's variations in average time length of surgical procedures compared with the database of the CDC National Nosocomial Infections Surveillance (NNIS) system. T-point baseline scores are not based on length of surgery as performed at the index hospital. The T-point number assigned to a procedure reflects a percentile (e.g., a T-point of 2 for hernia repair means that 75% of herniorrhaphies in the database were completed within 2 hours). This classification system looks at one variable and does not take into account other factors that may increase or decrease risk of surgical infection. Operative times that exceed any given T-point are associated with a greater chance of postoperative complications and risk of infection.

30. D: The NNIS Risk Index is scored from 0 (zero) to 3 (three) based on total points assigned as measured by four variables: wound classification (1 point if satisfies criteria for contaminated or dirty only); ASA preoperative score (1 point if ASA 3, 4, or 5); and T-point classification (1 point if procedure exceeds the T-point). Zero points are assigned if the patient has no risk factors. No single variable is assigned more than 1 point and none of the subscores are assigned a negative value. The correct answer is D, wherein 1 point is assigned for a preoperative ASA score of 3, 4, or 5 representing, respectively, severe systemic illness(es), life-endangering systemic disease(s), or a potentially preterminal state in which the patient is not expected to survive without surgical intercession.

31. C: Medical progress in this century moves in step with increased use of invasive testing and therapeutics. Despite their many benefits, devices must be regularly monitored for their associated risks and rates of infection. Specific and comparable measurements are useful for quality improvement, detection of unintended injury, and many other factors, included cost/benefit ratios and cost-effectiveness. To calculate overall infection rate for central line devices, determine the numerator, equal to the total number of infections: $2 + 1 + 4 = 7$. Divide by the denominator, calculated as the total number of device days: $48 + 20 + 72 = 140$. Thus, 7 infections $\div$ 140 = 0.05. To express this ratio or fraction per 1,000 device days, multiply $0.05 \times 1,000 = 50$, which is the overall hospital infection rate for this device.

32. D: Use the same calculation above to arrive at infection rates on each service.

Medical ICU: $2 \div 48 = 0.042 \times 1,000 = 42$

Surgical ICU: $1 \div 20 = 0.05 \times 1,000 = 50$

Oncology ward: $4 \div 72 = 0.056 \times 1,000 = 56$

Therefore, the oncology ward has the highest rate of infection expressed in device days. The 9 surgical ICU patients in this survey may not lend statistical significance to the result obtained but this service does not have the highest infection rate. The data obtained may still provide useful comparison information. These findings may alert the infection control team about variations in technique, patient selection, device preferences, or other early indicators that can be tracked or investigated in an effort to improve patient care.

33. B: Many different variables are used to determine statistical significance. No measurement is ideal nor should it be used without other supportive or challenging analyses. The P value is an accepted statistical method used to assess the likelihood that a statistical result resulted due to chance. A P value of 0.05 indicates a 5% probability that the result was caused by chance, or a 95% probability that it was not a random or chance event and is more likely a statistically sound occurrence. In statistics, P values less than (<) 0.05 are used to indicate higher probability of statistical significance. Statistical power can be increased by other variables, such as study design, number of subjects or events in the cohort studied, bias, and fulfillment of Hill's criteria. Here, the P values > 0.05 are not likely to fulfill statistical significance despite the larger cohort groups. Choices A and B have P values < 0.05, but choice A only measured 7 patients in an uncomplicated illness, leaving choice B as MOST likely to represent statistical validity.

34. A: Hospitals seeking to fulfill OSHA regulations for prevention of illnesses spread by bloodborne pathogenic microbes employ intermediate-level agents for disinfection, particularly in critical areas such as the emergency department, surgical suites (and related-use areas as in pre- and post-op recovery), and laboratories. Iodophors are examples of low-tier agents that kill most bacteria but may

not kill certain strains of fungi or viruses. Their lack of activity against resistant microbial strains and spores makes use of more effective agents imperative, especially in higher risk areas. A greater range of microbial kill or inactivation is seen with intermediate agents such as alcohol and sodium hypochlorite (bleach). This broader kill or inactivation range extends to vegetative organisms such as M. tuberculosis, viruses such as HBV and HIV, and fungi. High-level disinfectants additionally kill most bacterial, viral, and fungal strains, but may not fully eradicate areas, equipment, or surfaces contaminated by high concentrations of bacterial spores.

35. A: Flash sterilization is a method of heat sterilization that generally requires 3 to 10 minutes at 132°C to eradicate microbes, including most vegetative forms (ie, mycobacteria) and viruses, given appropriate and adequate pre-sterilization cleaning. These techniques are commonly used for reusable surgical equipment, especially when time and supply constraints demand rapid turnaround. Dry heat that uses oven-type equipment typically takes much longer and is not useful when sterilized materials are needed in short order. By definition, flash-sterilized items that have been appropriate precleaned will be rendered free of pathogens, including viruses, fungi, and vegetative microbes.

36. D: Decubiti develop in about one-third of patients with spinal cord injury. Given this high occurrence rate, decubitus ulcers present management issues that call for appropriate actions to prevent their development or hasten resolution in a timely manner by a well-educated clinical staff. Pressure and contamination combine to create a setting in which decubiti may develop. These factors underscore the role of active infection surveillance and interaction with clinical staff to ensure that patients are kept clean and that all available methods are employed (e.g., turning, special mattresses) to prevent excessive pressure and breaching of healthy, intact skin. Colonizing organisms are typically mixed, comprising aerobic and anaerobic flora. What may appear to be a small decubitus on the skin surface may instead represent more profound damage to subjacent soft tissue. Underlying osteomyelitis, or spread of infection to nearby bone, is commonly traced to a preexisting decubitus ulcer in these and other at-risk patient groups.

37. A: Surgical suite infection control practices must be known, assessed, and regularly revised to improve outcome measures. Routine sterilization procedures are preferable to flash sterilization, which may be incomplete because of inadequate precleaning, timing, or temperature considerations. Air exchange is also important, with at least 15 hourly air exchanges recommended, of which at least three should be using fresh air. Horizontal laminar air flow, air filtering, and positive pressure ventilation of hallways and areas adjacent to the surgical theatres should also be employed. Mechanical cleaning should be considered essential to proper postcleaning sterilization and should include daily wet vacuuming after the last procedure has been performed.

38. C: Nutrition service staff are an integral part of the health care team. They should be included in ongoing infection prevention and control strategies. They are permitted to deliver and remove trays from all patients with exception of those on precautions related to airborne pathogens. Although some institutions may choose disposables for their food service, paper and one-use items are not necessary. Food service staff should never move potentially contaminated items on a flip tray or surface so that food trays can be deposited. Instead, they must notify medical personnel so the item(s) can safely be disposed of and the tray or surface area properly cleansed. They should not remove trays that have been contaminated by medical equipment or body fluids, and should instead notify health care personnel rather than touch or cleanse an area themselves.

39. B: The FDA's MedWatch program provides a wealth of information related to drug and device recalls, safety updates, adverse event reporting, medical device reporting (MDR), and forms for detailing required events and voluntary case reports. Device-related incidents that require medical intervention

must be reported within 10 days. Facilities that use medical devices must issue MDR every 6 and 12 months. Although such facilities are encouraged to use MedWatch forms, they must also develop written procedures that detail what types of incidents must be reported using an MDR, how cases should be evaluated, and protocols for filing MDR. Records related to MDR must be kept for a minimum of 2 years.

40. D: Infection control coordinators are involved in occupational exposures to potential infectious agents that involve contact with skin, eyes, or mucous membranes, or a parenteral breach involving blood during execution of duties. IC staff consults and reports to hospital management regarding compliance with the institution's exposure control plan, appropriate interventions, investigations and education to help minimize risk for event recurrence, protect patient and staff, and strengthen prevention measures. OSHA standards regarding precautions for this type of procedure must be reviewed and documentation of the event must include compliance with such standards. Postexposure prophylaxis with HBIG may not be indicated in this case, regardless of perceived benefit of immediacy. The staff member should not be individually identified in communicating the incident to the rest of the staff, similar to patient privacy regulations. Exposure control plans do not dictate cessation of procedures that may be medically necessary while investigations are underway.

41. A: Participatory events such as hand washing contests that use materials designed to demonstrate technique efficacy in ridding hands of microbes are highly effective tools for staff education. As opposed to passive or didactic learning through posters, pamphlets, and other written materials, hands-on learning is a teaching tool associated with better penetration and retention of instructive material and, often, better recall and adherence to best-practices recommendations. While some medical personnel might say these activities are a waste of time, the effectiveness of these methods has been shown to be worthwhile. Students tend to be more receptive towards new information but they are not the only group likely to benefit from activities that reveal how each individual's habits may or may not be in step with regulations and best practices. All provider levels should be encouraged to improve handwashing habits through specific methods that can be easily learned and incorporated into new behaviors.

42. D: The infection control program annual summary is only as useful and the information it contains. Thus, specific information related to the goals and procedural guidelines of the institution's infection control program general plan must be included for maximal usefulness in future planning and assessment of adequacy of current procedures. Numerical and statistical examples, as applied to specific objectives such as surgical infection rates, are extremely helpful in this regard. Even if no incidents occurred, summaries must be filed with each goal and objective of the infection control program plan addressed. Occupational exposures are included in the exposure control plan and while they may be included in the infection control program annual summary, the report is not limited to these events. Financial summaries of cost-benefit and/or cost-effectiveness may be highlighted as part of the summary, but the document is not designed as an accounting or budgetary vehicle.

43. A: Even without ingrained old behaviors that may need to be revised, a new hospital presents its own set of challenges. Top priority in the development of an infection control program plan is to determine a profile of the institution (ie, patient base [sociodemographic profile, number of hospital beds], client needs [including that of patients, clinical staff, administrators, regulatory bodies, environmental engineers], size of health care personnel staff, types of services offered). While hardware and software may need to be upgraded at some point, initial efforts should not be directed towards costly endeavors without first assessing the strengths, limitations, needs, and expectations of the primary institution and its personnel. Assessment of client satisfaction is an important part of the final infection control program plan document but is not an initial priority, and will be incompletely assessed at a brief 30-day interval. Similarly, cost-benefit analysis comes into play once initial assessments are

underway and the IC officer/team begins to analyze problem areas or procedures in need of quality improvement.

44. A: Health care workers have specific responsibilities in overall infection control practices, particularly regarding their personal hygiene and habits. Nails, particularly when long or artificially enhanced, are a reservoir of potentially transmissible microbes, such as Staphylococcus, other skin flora, yeast, and pathogenic gram-negative rods such as Pseudomonas spp. Large numbers of potential pathogens can be recovered from the subungual areas of personnel who wear artificial nails, even in those who practice prudent handwashing techniques or use of surgical scrubs. While one-quarter inch length is the maximum recommended fingernail length, most bacteria are present within the first (most proximal) 1 mm of nail adjacent to subungual skin. Artificial nails present an infection hazard, even when fresh polish is applied daily. Chipped polish appears to harbor greater numbers of potentially infectious microbes, as can decorative flourishes such as sequins. Longer nails, whether natural or artificial, may predispose health care workers to injuring patients through inadvertent scratching or palpation that causes patient discomfort, whether physical or emotional. Longer nails may also tear through surgical gloves, potentially exposing health care workers to infectious materials. Because they interfere with precision during palpation, longer nails may interfere with proper clinical patient assessment, procedural performance, or handling of medical equipment.

45. C: The Food and Drug Administration (FDA) is the federal agency charged with the regulation of medications and medical devices. Their strict procedural guidelines outline regulations for preapproval of all prescription drugs and, through the Center for Devices and Radiologic Health (CDRH), medical devices. This also includes issuance of drug recalls and issues regarding safe reuse of medical equipment. Through the MedWatch program, FDA offers safety information and an avenue for reporting of adverse events. OSHA is a federal body whose regulatory powers include exposure to infectious agents in the workplace, as well as general and specific aspects of safety in the workplace. The Joint Commission is an accreditation body that sets standards for health care facilities, such as hospitals and outpatient surgical centers. The Centers for Disease Control and Prevention acts as a preventive and monitoring body that issues recommendation procedures for infectious disease control, hygiene, infection control practices, vaccination scheduling, and population-specific guidelines.

46. B: A Shewhart cycle is a problem-solving tool that employs four steps: Plan, Do, Check, Act. The method enables a systems approach to quality management. In this cycle, a process is identified and analyzed for problem or faulty processes, and root-cause analysis is done prior to developing a trial plan of action; followed by a check phase of analysis and determination of efficacy; and then to implementation and monitoring. Choices B to D are also used in performance improvement and educational efforts. A fishbone or Ishikawa diagram is used to help identify and illustrate cause and effect. A Pareto chart integrates two types of schematics: vertical bar graph and superimposed linear graph. Pareto charts help identify the greatest contributor to a given problem, as in 70% of all central lines that became infected were inserted by 10% of all residents. A flow chart is by definition a diagram or schematic that illustrates a process with directionality or flow, and input points to pictorially represent how a process unfolds or where problems and bottlenecks may occur.

47. D: Everyone wants handouts but they often go unused or filed next to the unread handout from last time. To be effective, handouts should not be distributed just as a presentation begins; an audience is likely to miss large parts of the presentation while flipping through the notes. Lengthy handouts with small font or smudged print, or those that incorporate difficult-to-read blocks of uninterrupted text are less likely to be considered useful. Bullet points are handy teaching tools, as are handouts that do not merely recapitulate the presentation material but highlight key points of the talk and underscore practical teaching points.

48. A: Compliance is calculated by measuring degree of fulfillment of a desired behavior or procedure. Traditionally expressed as a fraction or percentage, it is calculated by dividing the number of times a desired event occurs (numerator) by the total number of eligible procedures (denominator). When setting out to modify health care personnel behavior, it is important to observe, understand, and analyze in-place behaviors that may impede the desired behavioral change, whether by force of habit or conflicting rules, hierarchical concerns, and other factors. A useful technique is to demonstrate, reinforce, and then monitor as steps are taken to institute the desired change. Data may also be used to assess compliance, particularly when the effect of a desired change, such as the lowered infection rate in this case, can be easily measured and act as a surrogate marker for successful behavioral adaptation.

49. A: Policies and procedures for screening, vetting, and placing of candidate health care workers in medical facilities are developed along guidelines provided by four federal bodies: OSHA, CDC, the Joint Commission, and the American Hospital Association. The Joint Commission requires choice A, testing for drugs of abuse and background check, which may include criminal checks or some degree of financial/credit investigation as appropriate. OSHA recommends a tuberculin skin test performed in two stages. The standard Mantoux test involves intradermal purified protein derivative (PPD) injection. The injection site is read by a trained professional after 48 to 72 hours. TB testing is recommended to be performed at 1- and 3-week intervals to identify true negatives. A positive result necessitates a follow-up chest radiograph. While vaccination against hepatitis B is strongly recommended for health care workers, particularly those who work in higher risk areas, they are not required. However, employers may opt to engage nonimmune personnel in patient-care endeavors that involve lower risk of exposure to patients likely to harbor hepatitis B virus.

50. C: Herpetic whitlow is a type of herpes simplex infection of the skin that may manifest as blisters or vesicles on the finger, often at the tip. Virus may be shed from these lesions even when gloves are worn. Health care workers should be restricted from work until the lesions are fully healed. Latex allergy that manifests as dermatitis would qualify for work restriction but is noted in the example by history with no active lesions. This health care worker should be offered nonlatex gloves in his/her work station and advised of the need to have nonallergenic gloves on hand for situations where no nonallergenic gloves are immediately accessible. The nurse on ACE inhibitors with a new onset of nonproductive cough may be experiencing a common side effect of such drugs and does not require work restriction. However, health care workers with cough due to suspected viral or bacterial infection should be restricted from work until their symptoms clear.

Special Report: Additional Bonus Material

Due to our efforts to try to keep this book to a manageable length, we've created a link that will give you access to all of your additional bonus material.

Please visit http://www.mometrix.com/bonus948/cbic to access the information.